EAT
WELL,
LIVE
LONGER

EAT WELL, LIVE LONGER

Manual for a healthy heart

Edited by Marita Westberg

Translated by Larry Bertheaud

Illustrated by Sue Hunter

QUARTET BOOKS

LONDON · MELBOURNE · NEW YORK

Authors

General Nutrition: Dr Nancy Worcester
Diet and Heart Disease: Dr Richard Bruckdorfer
Recipes: Marita Westberg, Monica Kuhlin
and Larry Bertheaud in collaboration with Ann-Cathrine Björkman,
Sahlgren's Hospital, Gothenburg, Sweden

First published by Quartet Books Limited 1979
A member of the Namara Group
27 Goodge Street, London W1P 1FD

ISBN 0 7043 3219 1

Design by Mike Jarvis

Printed by Practical Publicity Ltd.

Contents

General Nutrition

by Dr Nancy Worcester

There is now a wider selection of foods available than ever before and seasonal foods can be purchased throughout the year. The average person now needs to allocate a smaller percentage of his/her budget to food in order to have an adequate diet. Moreover, each year scientists are discovering new facts about food composition and the role of food in the body. But what do these trends mean in terms of people's knowledge of food and the foods they are choosing to eat? Has a greater availability of foods and increased nutritional knowledge assured an adequate diet for everyone?

We only need to be reminded that over half the world's population has an inadequate diet to know that advanced technology and greater knowledge bear little relationship to what people actually eat. With 30 per cent of the world's population in rich, industrialized countries consuming (directly or indirectly) over half the world's cereals, it is obvious that it would take more than nutritional knowledge to enable hungry people in many areas to choose a satisfactory diet.

Good health, however, has not proved to be dependent upon the availability of an abundance of foods. The British were never so healthy as during the years of food rationing, and Americans who served years in Vietnam as prisoners of war returned home healthier (using blood pressure, diabetes, blood lipids and heart condition as indices of health) than the average American.

Many factors are at stake in determining our choice of diet, even if adequate foods are available and financial resources allow for their purchase.

Despite the fact that more is known and written about nutrition today than ever before, the general level of nutritional awareness is low and is not particularly influential in determining diet. A survey has shown that the husband has the greatest influence in determining a family's food habits, despite the fact that he is the family member least well informed about nutrition. Several studies have emphasized the need for better nutrition education. In a 1969 survey, only 6 per cent of respondents gave correct answers to nutritional questions. A more recent study (1975) of mothers of young children confirmed a general lack of nutritional awareness; only 5 per cent could answer two-thirds of the questions and most mothers overestimated their nutritional knowledge. Regardless of the fact that a national survey has established that most people are dependent upon their doctors for nutritional advice, medical schools continue to give minimal attention to nutrition in their curricula. It seems that what nutritional knowledge has been obtained is more often used to rationalize food choices already made than to influence these choices initially. Although many people will say they believe 'Brown bread is healthier than white bread', most of us choose to eat white bread.

An abundance of nutritional information is now appearing in bookshops, magazines and the media. How do we know which sources are reliable? This is difficult to determine because good, solid nutritional information does turn up in the most unexpected places (and vice versa). The following pages will serve as a brief summary of current nutritional knowledge, and any source deviating too drastically from this outline may be considered suspect. There is no magical food or nutrient which cures all ills, so we should be doubtful of any such claims. If we know something about one particular subject, it can be useful to evaluate the approach to that subject in a new book. For example, very little is known about the role of vitamin E in the human body, so any exaggerated claims about vitamin E may also be suspect in other respects. In general, sound nutritional sources will state that certain things are known, but that other things are still unknown. That is the state of nutrition today.

More than 3500 years ago Egyptians recommended ox liver for people who could not see at night, and by 1750 sailors were aware of the role of citrus fruits in preventing scurvy. But it has only been within the last fifty years that scientists have learned that it is the vitamin A in liver which is responsible for improved sight in dim light, and vitamin C which prevents scurvy. Nutrition has now shifted from the stage of discovering vitamins to the stage of trying to understand how these vitamins act at the biochemical level in the body's cells. To some extent, emphasis is shifting from determining the minimal requirements of certain nutrients to determining the role of large quantities of nutrients (e.g. the Megavitamin theories, and do large quantities of vitamin C help prevent the common cold?).

The relationship between diet and health has emerged as an important area of research. Few such relationships are fully understood and they remain controversial. A recent survey (1977) of members of the Nutrition Society (UK) illustrates how few nutritionists feel committed to various hypotheses relating to diet and disease. A large percentage of members answered that they were 'undecided' about each theory implicating a specific dietary component in the aetiology of a disease. This emphasizes the need for further research in order to fully appreciate the role diet may play in both preventative and curative medicine.

Requirements and Recommendations

A number of vitamins and minerals have now been identified and their role in the body is at least partially understood. From this information it has been possible to work out how much of each nutrient the body needs. Each individual requires different amounts of each nutrient, but there are now tables which give recommendations. These recommendations are based on wide individual differences, so are usually overestimates of what most individuals will actually require. (For most nutrients, it is safe to consume more than necessary, so this is appropriate, but overconsumption of energy/calories results in obesity, so calorie recommendations are based on 'average' need.) Recommendations serve as a useful guide for evaluating how effectively our diet is providing required nutrients. These tables are based on extrapolations from animal studies, human experimentation, and observations of human populations. Different groups have arrived at slightly different conclusions. The three most commonly used tables of recommendations are those of the Food and Agriculture Organization (USA), the National Research Council (USA), and the Department of Health and Social Services (UK). The British recommendations are given in Table 1.

Table 1: Recommended daily intake of nutrients
(Department of Health and Social Security, 1969)

Age ranges	Energy	Protein	Calcium	Iron	Vitamin A (retinol equivalent)	Thiamin	Riboflavin	Nicotinic acid equivalent	Vitamin C	Vitamin D
years	kcal	g	mg	mg	µg	mg	mg	mg	mg	µg
Infants										
Under 1	800	20	600	6	450	0.3	0.4	5	15	10
Children										
1	1,200	30	500	7	300	0.5	0.6	7	20	10
2	1,400	35	500	7	300	0.6	0.7	8	20	10
3-4	1,600	40	500	8	300	0.6	0.8	9	20	10
5-6	1,800	45	500	8	300	0.7	0.9	10	20	2.5
7-8	2,100	53	500	10	400	0.8	1.0	11	20	2.5
Males										
9-11	2,500	63	700	13	575	1.0	1.2	14	25	2.5
12-14	2,800	70	700	14	725	1.1	1.4	16	25	2.5
15-17	3,000	75	600	15	750	1.2	1.7	19	30	2.5
18-34 sedentary	2,700	68	500	10	750	1.1	1.7	18	30	2.5
18-34 moderately active	3,000	75	500	10	750	1.2	1.7	18	30	2.5
18-34 very active	3,600	90	500	10	750	1.4	1.7	18	30	2.5
35-64 sedentary	2,600	65	500	10	750	1.0	1.7	18	30	2.5
35-64 moderately active	2,900	73	500	10	750	1.2	1.7	18	30	2.5
35-64 very active	3,600	90	500	10	750	1.4	1.7	18	30	2.5
65-74	2,350	59	500	10	750	0.9	1.7	18	30	2.5
75 and over	2,100	53	500	10	750	0.8	1.7	18	30	2.5
Females										
9-11	2,300	58	700	13	575	0.9	1.2	13	25	2.5
12-14	2,300	58	700	14	725	0.9	1.4	16	25	2.5
15-17	2,300	58	600	15	750	0.9	1.4	16	30	2.5
18-54 most occupations	2,200	55	500	12	750	0.9	1.3	15	30	2.5
18-54 very active	2,500	63	500	12	750	1.0	1.3	15	30	2.5
55-74	2,050	51	500	10	750	0.8	1.3	15	30	2.5
75 and over	1,900	48	500	10	750	0.7	1.3	15	30	2.5
Pregnant, 2nd and 3rd										
trimesters	2,400	60	1,200	15	750	1.0	1.6	18	60	10
Lactating	2,700	68	1,200	15	1,200	1.1	1.8	21	60	10

Taken from Ministry of Agriculture, Fisheries and Food (1976); MANUAL OF NUTRITION (Her Majesty's Stationery Office, London).

The Basic Four Food Groups

Tables of recommendations are essential when it is necessary to evaluate a diet in specific detail. Fortunately, there are much easier ways of assessing diets on a day-to-day basis.

Even in this age of vitamin pills and tonics, most people still consume food as their source of nutrients. It is therefore reasonable to evaluate our diets in terms of the foods eaten, and possible to look up a specific food in a composition table, determine its nutrient content and compare this with the table's recommended daily intake. Such an exercise would show that an orange provides more than 100 per cent of the daily recommendation for vitamin C, but practically no protein. Similarly, a few ounces of cabbage provide more than 100 per cent of the recommended vitamin C intake, but little protein. In contrast, 4 oz of chicken provide nearly half of the protein recommendation, but no vitamin C. Based on the nutrients they contribute to the diet, foods can be divided into four basic groups: meats, fruits and vegetables, milk, and enriched breads and cereals.

Meats are valued for their protein content and contribute iron and B vitamins to the diet. Fruits and vegetables are reliable sources of vitamins and minerals, particularly vitamins A and C. The milk group provides protein, riboflavin, vitamin D and calcium. The enriched bread and cereal group is important for its protein, iron, B vitamins and energy content.

Table 2 summarizes the foods falling into each category and how many servings should be eaten daily from each group.

There is no 'basic four recommendation' for fats and oils, although this group is indispensable for supplying essential fatty acids, fat soluble vitamins and energy. Most diets contain sufficient amounts of the fats and oils and in fact most Western diets contain too much fat so there is no need to emphasize its inclusion in the diet. Similarly, there are no 'basic four recommendations' for sugars and sweets because these foodstuffs simply add 'empty calories' (calories not accompanied by valuable nutrients) to the diet and should be discouraged.

Table 2 : Basic Four Food Groups

FOOD GROUP	TYPES OF FOODS INCLUDED	DAILY RECOMMENDATION FOR ADULTS
MEAT (Protein group)	All meats, fish, eggs, nuts, pulses (legumes)	2 or more servings (1 serving = 2-3 oz meat, 1 egg, ½ cup pulses)
FRUITS and VEGETABLES	All fruits and vegetables	4 or more servings (1 serving = ½ cup or 1 piece) Eat 1 serving citrus fruit daily Eat dark green or deep yellow veg. every other day
MILK	Milk, cheese, yogurt	2 or more glasses
ENRICHED BREAD and CEREAL	Breads, cereals, rice, pasta, flours	4 or more servings (1 serving = 1 slice bread, 1 oz ready-to-eat cereal, ½-¾ cup cooked cereal or pasta)

The Six Basic Nutrients

Let us now take a more detailed look at our knowledge of the nutrients and their roles in the body.

Most foods are complex mixtures of many nutrients which are essential for enabling the body to survive and function. All nutrients can be categorized into one of the following six classes:

1 Water
2 Carbohydrates
3 Fats
4 Proteins
5 Vitamins
6 Minerals

1 Water

Water, which receives the least attention, is the most important nutrient. The body will succumb to water deprivation sooner than to starvation, since water is involved in nearly every body process. Where drinking water is accessible, this nutrient is readily available, but there are still parts of the world where drinking water is inaccessible.

2 Carbohydrates

Three groups of nutrients are classified as carbohydrates: starches, sugars, and cellulose and related materials. The body needs energy for brain functioning, maintenance of body temperature, utilization of foods, and body movements. The carbohydrates provide this energy. Pure carbohydrate provides the body with approximately 4 kilocalories (4 calories) per gram (or 1 ounce of carbohydrate = 112 kilocalories. Kilocalories/calories are simply a measurement of the energy value of foods). If carbohydrate consumption is greater than the body's requirement, the body turns the carbohydrate into fat and stores it. Most of us have made our own observations of bread and potatoes turning into body fat!

Throughout the world, carbohydrates play a major role in the diet because they are readily available, cost less than other foods, and store more easily. In Third World countries carbohydrates often make up 90 per cent of the diet, in contrast to providing only 40 per cent of the calories in most Western diets.

One hundred and fifty years ago carbohydrates were almost entirely consumed as starches, in the form of breads, cereals, potatoes, legumes (pulses), rice and pasta. Since then, sugar has drastically replaced starch in the diet. The average annual sugar consumption was 25 lb in 1850 compared with 120 lb in 1950, and nutritionists are concerned about this trend. Starch foods usually carry other nutrients with them, whereas sugars are only a source of energy. Extra energy consumption can easily lead to obesity, and for children, particularly, it is dangerous for sugar to replace more nutritional foods in the diet. There is general agreement that dental caries is related to a high sugar intake and there is growing interest in whether increased sugar consumption is related to the increased prevalence of heart disease, diabetes and high blood pressure (*see* next chapter).

Until recently, little attention has been focused on the third group of carbohydrates: cellulose and related materials (now referred to as dietary fibre or roughage). Dietary fibre has previously been considered almost as a food impurity because the body is unable to derive any nutritional value from it and it simply passes through the body.

It has now been noted, however, that societies with a high fibre diet do not have many of the diseases (large intestine diseases such as diverticulosis and large bowel cancer, appendicitis, obesity, gall bladder disease, heart disease, and diabetes) prevalent in Western societies consuming a low-fibre diet. This has prompted nutritionists to examine the role fibre may play in promoting health. Fibre is known to contribute bulk to the diet and food passes through the system more quickly on a high-fibre diet. Fibre influences the absorption of nutrients and is believed to help remove harmful substances from the body.

Whole grain cereals and flours, potatoes, vegetables, legumes (pulses), nuts and fruits are the primary sources of dietary fibre. An average Western diet contains only 4.2 grams of crude fibre per day, compared with 20 grams per day in vegetarian diets or 25 grams per day in that of an average African peasant. There is now sufficient evidence to suggest that an increase in dietary fibre may be beneficial and should be encouraged.

3   Fats

Fats provide more than 40 per cent of the total energy in many Western diets in contrast with providing only 15 per cent of the energy in diets in poorer countries. Only a third of the fat consumed is 'visible' fat (e.g. butter, margarine and oils). Meats, milk, cheese, eggs, biscuits and cakes are largely responsible for the high fat intake in Western diets.

Fats are a compact source of energy, containing 9 kilocalories (9 calories) per gram (250 kcal/ounce) compared with approximately 4 kilocalories per gram (112 kcal/ounce) from proteins and carbohydrates. Thus, fats provide energy in the diet without adding excess bulk. Fats slow the emptying time of the stomach and contribute to the feeling of fullness after a meal. Most people find a low-fat diet to be lacking in interest as fats contribute largely to the palatability, texture and taste of foods.

The optimum level of fat in the diet is not known. Fats are a source of the fat soluble vitamins A, D, E and K, and contain the essential fatty acids (EFA). Even the poorest diets supply sufficient essential fatty acids, so a fat deficiency *per se* is not a problem in human diets. (*See* the next chapter for a fuller discussion of fats in the diet.)

4   Protein

Body proteins can only be made from proteins supplied by the diet, so it is essential that the diet regularly supplies an adequate quantity. Although the body requires extra protein in periods of growth and repair (i.e. growing children, pregnant and lactating women, and in conditions of illness and stress) even mature adults need protein to cover the breakdown and replacement of body proteins which takes place daily throughout our lifetime. In addition to their role in making new cells for growth, maintenance and repair, proteins are required for the synthesis of special protein compounds (i.e. antibodies, enzymes, hormones) which regulate body processes. Protein can be used to provide energy for the body (4 kilocalories/gram) (112 kilocalories/ounce) if the diet does not supply sufficient energy from other sources.

Many foods contain protein, and cultures differ greatly in their sources of dietary protein. In typical Western diets, we derive over a quarter of our protein from the meat group, and a quarter from the breads, flours, and cereals group. One-fifth of our protein comes from milk. Cheese, fish, eggs, potatoes and other vegetables also contribute to the protein content of our diet.

Western diets also differ greatly from those of the Third World in the level of protein intake. It is known that adults can remain healthy on diets containing far lower amounts of protein than those usually consumed, and in most Western diets protein intake is 50 per cent higher than the recommended level. The body can adapt to widely different levels of dietary protein. Excess protein offers no biological advantage and is usually an expensive energy source.

Proteins are made up of many smaller units, the amino-acids, joined together. There are twenty-two amino-acids which can be joined together in thousands of different combinations to make specific proteins. Eight of these must be supplied by the diet and are thus referred to as the essential amino-acids. The body can make the remaining fourteen (non-essential) amino-acids once the essential amino-acids have been supplied.

Proteins are evaluated in terms of whether they supply the essential amino-acids in a ratio which can be used efficiently by the body. If a protein is greatly lacking in one (the limiting) amino-acid, the body cannot use all of the other amino-acids supplied by that protein. Some protein foods (milk and eggs) have amino-acid patterns similar to the human body and these proteins are used very efficiently. In a mixed meal where several protein foods are eaten simultaneously, the limiting amino-acid of one food will compensate for or complement the limiting amino-acid of another, so the proteins from both can be used efficiently. If vegetable proteins are eaten on their own, they are not as efficient as animal proteins, but in combinations vegetables can be excellent sources of protein. Good combinations are:

grains + pulses (legumes)
grains + milk products
nuts + pulses (legumes)

5 Vitamins

The vitamins are a group of unrelated organic (carbon-containing) chemicals. The body requires many unique chemicals in order to carry out the processes required for growth and maintenance of life; it can make most of its own chemicals, but the vitamins are a special group which the body cannot make and so the diet must supply. Animals differ as to which vitamins must be supplied by the diet. For example, humans, guinea pigs and monkeys must have vitamin C supplied daily in the diet but most other animals can make their own. Vitamins do not supply energy (calories) to the body.

Vitamins are required in extremely small amounts, which is convenient since they occur naturally in foods in small quantities. A 4-oz orange contains more than the recommended daily intake of vitamin C and yet the orange only contains one part vitamin C (ascorbic acid) for every 2500 parts orange! Thirty mg (the recommended daily intake of vitamin C) is barely visible when weighed out in a small tube and most of the other vitamins are required in even smaller quantities.

The important roles played by vitamins in the body are in no way proportional to the minute quantities in which they are required. Most of them act as catalysts, speeding up chemical reactions required by the body. Each vitamin functions in a very specific way or ways (see Table 3), and specific deficiencies occur when it is not present in the necessary quantity.

Table 3.   The Vitamins

VITAMIN	FUNCTIONS	DEFICIENCY	SOURCES	STABILITY	OTHER COMMENTS
FAT SOLUBLE VITAMINS					
VITAMIN A	1. Prevention of night blindness 2. Involved in colour vision 3. Essential for formation & maintenance of cells lining & covering body 4. Essential for normal growth	eye lesions or complete blindness	fish oils dairy prod. liver kidney eggs green & yellow veg.	fairly stable sometimes destroyed by high-temp. frying	excessive intake possible with synthetic vitamins
VITAMIN D 'The Sunshine Vitamin'	Required for the body to absorb calcium & phosphorous & to use these for bone formation, growth & maintenance	rickets (failure of growing bones to calcify) osteomalacia (loss of calcium from bones)	oils fish eggs dairy prod. breads cereals	stable	in a sunny climate, vit. D does not need to be supplied by diet
VITAMIN E	Not fully known Functions as an antioxidant so protects such compounds as vitamins A, C & polyunsaturated fatty acids	sometimes in premature infants	almost all foods, esp. veg. oils cereal germ leafy veg. milk eggs		requirement influenced by other factors in the diet
VITAMIN K	Performs essential role in blood coagulation	haemorrhagic (bleeding) disease of newborn or as a secondary disease	green leafy veg. peas cereals made in the body		
WATER SOLUBLE VITAMINS					
VITAMIN C Ascorbic acid	1. Used for building & maintaining bones & connective tissue 2. Essential for blood vessels 3. Plays a role in wound healing	scurvy (bleeding in into joints & from gums)	fruits, esp. citrus potatoes other veg.	most fragile vitamin- destroyed by heat, air, light, copper & iron very soluble in water	

VITAMIN	FUNCTIONS	DEFICIENCY	SOURCES	STABILITY	OTHER COMMENTS
THE 'B' VITAMINS					
VITAMIN B$_1$ Thiamin	1. Involved in carbohydrate & fat metabolism 2. Required for nerve functioning	beri-beri (inflamed nerves, loss of muscle power, heart failure)	milk peanuts liver pork eggs, veg. fruit	destroyed by high temp. alkali, very soluble in water	
VITAMIN B$_2$ Riboflavin	Involved in protein, fat, & carbohydrate metabolism	seldom occurs by itself (usually with other B deficiencies)	milk green veg. fish, eggs meat, esp. liver and kidney	destroyed by light very soluble in water	
NIACIN	Involved in protein, fat & carbohydrate metabolism	pellegra (affects skin, mucous membranes & nerves)	meat, esp. liver peanuts pulsus (legumes) fish, mushrooms whole grain cereals	very soluble in water	
VITAMIN B$_6$ Pyridoxine	Involved in protein metabolism & haemoglobin formation		meats fish eggs whole cereals		
FOLIC ACID		megoblastic anaemia	liver pulses (legumes) bread green leafy veg.	very soluble in water	
VITAMIN B$_{12}$		pernicious anaemia	only in animal foods esp. liver eggs, cheese milk, meat fish	soluble in water	most recent (1948) vitamin isolated

The functions fulfilled by vitamins were recognized long before they were identified. Early experiments demonstrated that rats did not grow properly without 'Factor A', but it was many years before the specific chemicals — retinol and related compounds — were identified as being responsible for vitamin A activity. The group originally referred to as 'vitamin B' turned out to comprise several specific vitamins, including B$_1$ (thiamine), B$_2$ (riboflavin), nicotinic acid, B$_6$ (pyridoxine), folic acid, pantothenic acid and biotin. These vitamins are still thought of as a group because they tend to occur in the same foods and are all involved in the utilization of energy. The most recently (1948) identified vitamin, B$_{12}$, is now known to be cyanocabalamin, but is still referred to as B$_{12}$ for fairly obvious reasons!

Vitamins are classified as either fat soluble or water soluble. The fat soluble vitamins A, D, E and K are stored in the fat of the body and do not therefore need to be supplied every day. They are often found in fatty foods (margarine, butter, oils, oily fish, dairy products). In contrast, the water soluble vitamins, Bs and C, are not stored in the body and must be supplied regularly.

It has been accepted in the past that the body needs a certain amount of each vitamin and that anything supplied in excess of that amount will be neither a help nor hindrance. This idea is now a controversial issue, and popular writers are making a fortune from books suggesting that large quantities of certain vitamins will promote youthfulness, virility and other *supposedly* desirable characteristics. Even respected scientisists have advocated using large quantities of vitamins for the preservation of good health and the treatment of disease. Best known of these advocates is Linus Pauling (Nobel Chemistry and Peace Prize winner) who proposes that large quantities of vitamin C will prevent the common cold. Such ideas merit further investigation, but we need to be careful in encouraging the public to take massive quantities of vitamins. When eating natural foods, with the exception of polar bear oil which contains an excessive amount of vitamin A, it is impossible to get too much of any vitamin, but it *is* possible to take too much in the concentrated, synthetic form. Although it is generally accepted that extra water soluble vitamins will simply be 'washed out of the system' (expensive urine!), it is not actually known how the body adjusts to long term intakes of large quantities. Since fat soluble vitamins are stored by the body, excessively large doses of these are dangerous and may even cause death. In the USA there has been much debate as to whether the fat soluble synthetic vitamins should be classified as prescription drugs so that the general public cannot abuse their use.

The vitamin content of foods is at its peak in the fresh foods eaten in the raw state. Some vitamins, particularly those which are water soluble, are quite fragile and easily destroyed, so any method of preparation may reduce the nutrient content. However, with some thought, the vitamin loss in preparation can be kept to a minimum. In general, foods should be cooked for as brief a time as possible, at low temperatures, and in a minimal quantity of liquid. Cooking liquid should be saved, as it will be full of nutrients, and can be consumed in an appropriate way, i.e. in soup making. Foods should be prepared and served as quickly as possible because both advance soaking and 'keeping warm' destroy some vitamins. The outer leaves and the part of the vegetable near the skin are usually vitamin richest, so eating these parts should be encouraged. Bicarbonate of soda destroys vitamins B and C so should not be added to cooking water. There is less loss of vitamins if vegetables are cut into large pieces with smaller surface area than in small pieces. Since the freezing process has little effect on nutrient content, foods picked at their peak and frozen are often nutritionally superior to those shipped from the countryside to the town and and stored for some time before being sold as 'fresh foods'.

6 Minerals

The sixth group of nutrients is the minerals, a group of inorganic chemicals required by the body and comprising 4 per cent of its composition. (The other 96 per cent is water, fat, protein and carbohydrate.) Like vitamins, minerals do not supply energy (calories) to the body.

The minerals function in two ways, as regulatory and as building substances. As structural components in hard substances (bones and teeth), as constituents in soft tissues (muscles and nervous tissues), and as components in specific chemicals (hormones, enzymes), the minerals exhibit their role as building substances. As regulators, the minerals are involved in maintaining water balance and acid-base balance, and in initiating essential reactions.

Table 4. The Minerals

MINERAL	FUNCTIONS	SOURCES	OTHER COMMENTS
CALCIUM	1. Essential for growth & maintenance of bone & teeth 2. Required for blood clot formation 3. Required for heart beat 4. Required for muscle contraction 5. Required for nerve functioning	milk, milk prod. green leafy vegetables small fish bones, fortified cereals	deficiency = bone & teeth decalcify only 20-50% absorbed from most foods
CHLORIDE	1. Balancing mechanism in blood 2. Provides acidity (HC1) of stomach for digestion	table salt meat, eggs milk	
IODINE	Essential component of hormone (thyroxine) for energy regulation	foods grown in iodine rich soil	deficiency = goitre & cretinism
IRON	Component of haemoglobin & myoglobin (oxygen carriers in blood & muscle)	organ meats meats seafood green leafy veg. egg yolk nuts iron enriched foods	deficiency = anaemia only 5-30% absorbed from most foods
MAGNESIUM	1. Involved in 100s of metabolic reactions 2. Required for nerve impulse conduction	in most foods especially green leafy veg., cereals, nuts, seafood, cocoa	
PHOSPHORUS	1. Used in teeth & bone formation 2. Plays vital role in carbohydrate, fat, & protein metabolism 3. Helps regulate blood acidity	fruits veg. meats	

MINERAL	FUNCTIONS	SOURCES	OTHER COMMENTS
POTASSIUM	1. Required for carbohydrate, protein metabolism 2. Required for nerve impulse conduction 3. Helps maintain acid-base balance	most foods	
SODIUM	1. Helps regulate body fluids 2. Helps maintain body acidity 3. Required for nerve impulse conduction 4. Involved in muscle conduction	most foods table salt processed foods	miners' cramp = excessive loss through perspiration high salt intake may be related to high blood pressure

Table 4 summarizes information about the minerals occurring in the largest quantities in the body. On a typical Western diet, we probably need to be most concerned that our diet should supply adequate iron and calcium. Only a part of the calcium and iron in foods is actually absorbed and used by the body, so it is necessary for the diet to supply somewhat more than the body requires. However, the recommendation tables (Table 1) already take this limited absorption into consideration so we do *not* need to supply more than is recommended. Certain factors are known to increase or decrease the absorption of calcium and iron from foods (*see* section on interrelationships). Many foods, particularly cereal products, are now enriched with calcium and iron as a matter of routine, so deficiencies are not the problem they could be in a society unaware of the need to supply these nutrients in the diet.

The body does partially compensate for poor diets in that iron absorption is most efficient when iron is most needed, and the body also seems to adjust to low calcium intakes. However, iron deficiency anaemia is still one of the world's most common nutritional problems, and this is even so in Western women of childbearing age. Women's diets need to be more iron-concentrated (more iron supplied by less calorific foods) than those of men. Iron supplied by animal foods is somewhat more efficiently absorbed than that supplied by vegetable sources, but vegetarian diets can supply an adequate iron intake.

With the possible exceptions of iron and calcium, our ordinary diets supply sufficient quantities of the minerals in the small amounts needed by the body. In fact, we are becoming increasingly aware that our modern lifestyles — consuming many processed foods, living in polluted environments — may provide too many minerals. High salt (sodium) intake is probably related to high blood pressure. Recent scares about mercury poisoning from fish and excess lead in processed foods and city environments, are indications of many issues which may need to be resolved about our over-exposure to minerals.

Techniques are increasingly available to unravel some of the mysteries regarding those minerals which are either required in very small amounts or are dangerous in very small quantities. The group referred to as trace elements, because they are present in foods and body tissues in minute amounts, includes iodine, fluorine, zinc, copper, cobalt, manganese, selenium, chromium, molybdenum, cadmium, lead, mercury, arsenic, lithium, boron, tin, vanadium, nickel, silicon and aluminium. The role, if any, of many of these trace elements is not yet known. Very sophisticated instruments and techniques are required, and increasingly available, to measure the elements and to create a deficiency in experimental animals.

Interrelationships between Nutrients

We have now considered in some detail our knowledge of the specific nutrients. However, it is essential to remember that no nutrient is consumed in isolation from another. All foods are made up of a number of nutrients which nature has packaged together, and we usually consume several foodstuffs simultaneously. Even if we were to try living on a totally synthetic diet, we would still be consuming a mixture of nutrients. The combinations in which we choose to consume our nutrients influence their interaction and how our bodies make use of them.

This interaction of one nutrient with another has made it very difficult for nutritionists to elucidate information about specific nutrients, to determine their functions and to establish recommended intakes.

Vitamin E stands out as an obvious example of a nutrient about which our knowledge is limited because of its complex interaction with several others. Selenium, a trace mineral, is known to reduce the requirement for vitamin E, but in experimental animals selenium prevents some but not all signs of vitamin E deficiency. Polyunsaturated fatty acids increase the requirement for vitamin E, a fact worth noting when the replacement of dietary saturated fats with polyunsaturated fats is advocated. Any such drastic change in the diet will probably influence requirements, and it has been suggested that high saturated-fat diets increase the requirement for essential fatty acids (found in the polyunsaturated fatty acids).

Little is known about the long-term effects of massive doses of vitamin C, although it has been suggested that such doses could increase the requirements for other nutrients, i.e. vitamin B_{12}. It is even more likely that prolonged use of large doses of vitamin C would increase the minimal requirement of the body for this vitamin for scurvy prevention. Other factors in our diet and environment may also influence our vitamin C requirement. For example, if the suggestion that smokers have an increased vitamin C requirement is true, it is easy to postulate that people living in polluted cities may require more vitamin C than their country cousins.

Proteins, fats and carbohydrates are all capable of providing energy for the body, but only proteins can be used to make new body proteins. If the diet does not provide sufficient fat and carbohydrate to fulfil energy requirements, then the protein will be burned up for energy instead of being used for protein synthesis. Carbohydrates are thus valued for their 'protein sparing action'.

The B vitamins are needed to utilize the energy from foods, hence their requirement is related to food intake. And high energy diet will increase the B requirement.

One of the amino-acids, tryptophan, can be converted in the body to the vitamin nicotinic acid. Consequently, a diet high in tryptophan will reduce the nicotinic acid requirement. This is taken into consideration in the recommendation table (Table 1) where the requirement for nicotinic acid is given in terms of 'equivalents' (1 nicotinic acid equivalent = 1 mg nicotinic acid = 60 mg tryptophan.)

Factors in the diet can also influence the efficiency with which the body uses the nutrients contained in foods. In the average diet, only 5-30 per cent of the iron and 20-50 per cent of the calcium in food is absorbed and used, but many factors can decrease or increase the efficiency of calcium and iron absorption. Vitamin D, proteins and lactose (milk sugar) all increase calcium absorption. Dairy products contain not only calcium, but also all three factors necessary to encourage its absorption. Oxalic acid (present in some fruits and vegetables) and fats decrease calcium absorption. Vitamin C increases iron absorption whereas the phosphate in egg yolk decreases this process. Phytic acid (phytate) present in the bran layers of grain decreases the absorption of both calcium and iron. There is much more phytic acid in wholemeal or brown bread than in white bread, so the 'brown vs white bread' controversy is more complicated than many wholemeal advocates appreciate.

Nutritional Problems and Vulnerable Groups

It is a sad reflection on the world today that we are faced with two distinct nutritional problems; malnutrition and over-nutrition.

Malnutrition — a lack of sufficient quantities of nutrients to ensure adequate health — is a major problem in almost every Third World country. Twenty per cent of the populations in the Middle East, Africa and Asia suffer from iron deficiency anaemia. Vitamin A deficiency, often resulting in blindness, still affects more than 20,000 children a year in Arabia, Africa and Latin America. Famines continue to 'happen' despite modern technology which should be able to prevent them, and people starve to death or die because of their over-susceptibility to infection, more through a lack of money to pay for food than because of its actual unavailability.

The most serious nutritional problem, still prevalent in many parts of the world, is protein-energy malnutrition (PEM) in which neither protein nor energy is supplied in adequate quantities. In some countries, over 70 per cent of the pre-school children are affected and many children die before the age of five. Those who survive may suffer mental retardation for the rest of their lives. Breast milk is the best source of nutrients for an infant, and even the most malnourished mother miraculously seems able to produce adequate milk for her baby. This fact should ensure most babies a decent start in life even in the worst economic conditions. However, commercial firms have recently started marketing artificial milks to mothers in Third World countries. These women cannot afford to buy the artificial milk in adequate quantities and often do not have adequate sanitary conditions for its preparation. Tragically, this development has greatly increased the incidence of protein-energy malnutrition while making a few milk companies very rich.

In contrast, over-nutrition — eating too much of the wrong foods — is the *biggest* nutritional problem in most Western countries. Obesity, heart disease, diabetes and bowel diseases are all at least partially related to our patterns of over-consumption (*see* next chapter).

Even within our affluent societies, nutritional deficiency diseases do exist. Because of special requirements and circumstances, certain groups of the population are most vulnerable to nutritional problems. Special ethnic and cultural groups probably pose a nutritional challenge for every society. In Britain, there is increasing awareness of rickets in Asian children who consume a diet which would have been sufficient in vitamin D in a sunny climate. Vitamin D is formed by sunshine from a compound in the body, so the need for dietary vitamin D is greatly reduced in sunny climates. In England, a country known to suffer from sun deficiency, the typical Asian diet may result in vitamin D deficiency. In the United States, the American Indian and migrant workers and their families suffer severe nutritional problems directly related to their appalling economic and social positions. Most of the nutritional conditions we have just listed as typical in the Third World are also problems for these communities in the midst of affluent America.

Pregnancy and lactation (breast feeding) increase the requirements of the body for many nutrients (*see* Table 1). Extra milk, meats, liver and fortified cereals should be encouraged to meet these additional needs. An adequate diet is essential at this time to ensure good health for both mother and foetus. The incidence of miscarriage, prematurity, and still birth are much more frequent in malnourished women than in those with an adequate diet.

Malnutrition most often affects the elderly members of the population. In Britain, it has been suggested that 3 per cent of the elderly suffer from overt malnutrition while a much larger number probably suffer from subclinical malnutrition. Diets for the elderly must be more vitamin and mineral concentrated than those for other sections of the population, simply because the requirements for the vitamins and minerals remain the same (or increase due to poor absorption, illness etc.) while the energy/calorie requirement is 20-30 per cent lower (due to relative lack of activity). Obesity is common in older people who do not reduce their food intake and often complicates other conditions such as arthritis and rheumatic disease. Vitamin (folic acid, vitamin C, vitamin D, thiamine) and iron deficiencies are common in older people who simply reduce their food intake without watching the nutrient intake. Easy-to-prepare, low-calorie, high-nutritional foods are essential for the elderly. Milk and dairy products, enriched breads and cereals, frozen vegetables and minced meats are appropriate. Meals on Wheels and Community Day Clubs are providing an invaluable nutritional and social contribution to the life of the elderly, and thus to the community. More products especially designed for the tastes, nutritional requirements and limited financial resources of the elderly must be made available to minimize the nutritional problems in this ever increasing section of the population.

Let us now focus on heart diseases, one of those diseases we mentioned as being at least partially related to our patterns of over-consumption.

Diet and Heart Disease

by Dr Richard Bruckdorfer

We all know of friends or relatives who have been severely afflicted, often fatally, by the modern scourge known as coronary heart disease and its related disorders. Many people regard these premature deaths or disabilities with resignation. The usual reaction is to murmur explanations based on the victim's worried life or family history.

Only a small minority have made special efforts to prevent the occurrence of these diseases. Such people are often armed with strong ideas on 'natural' foods or the value of physical exercise. For the less committed majority there is often only uncertainty or bewilderment after reading the sporadic articles in the press which describe the views of the many experts in the field. This advice, which is sometimes contradictory, reflects the variety of opinions held by medical scientists on the origins of heart disease and the best methods of preventing it.

It is widely held that we are dealing with a disease caused by a variety of factors, but sometimes experts cannot resist emphasizing their own pet theory to the exclusion of others. Nevertheless, some views have dominated medical opinion as we shall discuss below. Fortunately, more concerted attempts have been made to collate current opinions and to present these concisely. Although popular books (of rather variable value) have been written, these tend to be read by the aware or the anxious, and have not reached the mass of the population.

Food manufacturers have in a few instances taken heed of these problems, especially if their product is considered healthful by the current theories. There is a silent but fierce battle between various sections of the food industry through investment in research programmes to deflect blame from particular foods which may be in question.

From this confusion, we believe that it is possible to take a consensus of the expert advice and to present a comprehensive programme both on diet and the non-dietary factors, which can be a platform on which the majority of experts agree even though some may not see any value in the inclusion or exclusion of particular items. Such programmes are in existence in some countries, e.g. United States and Norway, and in Britain the report of the Joint Working Party of the Royal College of Physicians and the British Cardiac Society was printed in the *Journal of the Royal College of Physicians of London*. This journal is likely to be read by the medical profession and other interested parties, but it seems unlikely that its recommendations will quickly, if ever, disseminate to the population as a whole. Clearly a massive drive, beginning in schools or in factory or office canteens, is required to have an impact.

There is a need to give practical advice which will cause the least possible change to traditional patterns of eating or other activities. This is a sharp lesson learned from nutritional programmes concerning under-nutrition in the Third World. It is also essential that the changes should be permanent and not a seven-day wonder. We should not adopt the idea that there is a single factor — a panacea — which is the key food component in these diseases, and that all that has to be done is to identify it and simply eliminate it from our diets.

With heart disease we are faced with a chronic abnormality of our body chemistry, which takes years to manifest itself. It is the slowness of these changes which makes it so difficult to study and determine the causatory factors. Nevertheless the complexity of the changes does encourage the view that many single factors can interact with each other and influence the course of disease. With these guidelines we can feel less bewildered and plan a reasonable diet based on the available information.

Before we consider the details, perhaps it would be worth mentioning the subject of 'natural' foods, since a substantial minority believe that the consumption of unwholesome foods, adulterated by food manufacturers, lies at the root of our modern health problems. Let us, however, point out that it is easy to eat a combination of 'natural' foods, untouched by the manufacturer, which is quite unsatisfactory. What we must consider is the best *combination* of available foods, whether natural or manufactured, to rid us of the disabilities of heart disease.

It is difficult to define the natural human diet, because it has changed radically even during our pre-industrial era. There is a popular view of early man as a hunter of large animals and of meat as a principal component of our natural diet. It is recognized that the 'gathering' of roots, seeds, nuts and fruit was a more consistent source of food and largely carried out by women. The advent of agriculture, selection of seeds, clearing of land, domestication of animals and preservation and manufacture of foods from agricultural produce came at a later stage of human development. The medicine of the Greeks and later of Galen had a profound influence on European diets. In the Middle Ages, vegetables and fruit were generally spurned as origins of bowel problems. Consequently land scurvy was prevalent as well as the more renowned outbreaks at sea.

In industrialized society remarkable changes have been brought about. We have a legacy of poverty and bad food in the nineteenth century in part due to food adulteration, poverty, poor public health and the difficulties of transport and preservation of food. It is this problem of preservation which, coupled with the manufacture of new foods of dubious value, gives rise to concern in a better informed health conscious world. The types of disease which now afflict us are different, but this is not totally attributable to our modern diet because so many other changes have occurred. It seems highly unlikely that we will return to a hunter/gatherer existence with such a huge global population or that all forms of food manufacture will be discontinued in order to be completely natural.

There are good reasons for giving our dietary habits a full examination, as you will see. First of all, let us briefly examine the development of this disease of the arteries and then consider how our food and other factors affect it.

What Happens to Your Arteries in Coronary Heart Disease?

The simple answer to this question is that they get blocked, which prevents the supply of blood to the heart and thus deprives it of essential oxygen and nutrients. This involves a blockage of one or more of the coronary arteries supplying the heart muscles (which become severely damaged) and can cause death if the damage is extensive. Arteries supplying the brain can also be affected, bringing about a stroke, and other organs can be impaired.

The blockage is caused by a narrowing of the central tube or lumen of the artery through which the blood is pumped. In addition, blood clots often lodge in the constricted parts. These two abnormal processes have attracted the attention of research scientists who study them in order to seek clues as to the origin of the disease. There is as yet no agreement on the sequence of events leading to the thickening of the artery walls (arteriosclerosis).

The predominant view is that the initial response is due to local damage from a variety of agents (including high levels of blood fats), which leads to changes in the permeability of the arterial walls and the multiplication of cells in underlying tissues. However, in the process, fats present in the blood (see below) are deposited in the artery wall and one in particular, cholesterol, accumulates there because it cannot be degraded at that site. Fatty streaks which are so formed can be observed in infants, but there is doubt as to their association with later lesions in adults. Fatty deposits associated with fibrin, a blood protein, can frequently be observed in autopsies of young men who have died from other causes. There is also evidence that small clots of blood or thrombi adhere to these abnormal regions. There may be several episodes of deposition and cell multiplication leading up to middle age, which narrow the affected arteries but do not cause any clinical problems. These fibrous/fatty lesions can with time ulcerate and rupture, leading to serious clot formation and local arterial blockage and a heart attack. Severe constriction of the coronary arteries can lead to angina pains, again because of cramps in the heart muscle. Older lesions sometimes become encased with deposits of calcium salts.

A more recent 'monoclonal' theory of arterial abnormality suggests that the whole sequence of events begins with one or more cells being mutated by a variety of agents and multiplying like cancer cells. Although this idea has not received widespread acceptance, it warrants further investigation.

There are many difficulties in studying the causes of this disease because of the protracted length of its development and the ethical problems of using human subjects. Useful results can be obtained from animal experiments, but these must be regarded with caution because animals are different from humans in many respects. Other evidence can be obtained from trends in whole populations, with the study of mortality from heart disease in relation to their measurable attributes, habits and activities. This we call epidemiology. We can now begin to examine briefly the factors which are alleged to play a part in the development of heart disease and try to reach some useful conclusions.

Who is at Risk?

This is a difficult question with no simple answer. It is not possible to say that any indvidual runs no risk of sustaining a heart attack, just that the likelihood is low or very low. In the other direction, only high risk can be predicted, except perhaps in the case of recognizable genetic defects where predictions of near certainty can be made. What can be said is that broadly speaking an inhabitant of an industrialized country stands a high risk of a clinical manifestation of the disease, whereas the condition is almost unknown in some poor Third World countries. This can be shown from the morbidity and mortality statistics collected by epidemiologists. It can be seen from the mortality statistics for England and Wales that coronary heart disease and related disorders are the cause of death for 52 per cent of men in the age range 45 to 54 years and 41 per cent of all deaths in 35- to 44-year old men (Fig. 1). Most of these deaths are due to coronary heart disease itself. For women, who have a lower mortality from all causes, coronary heart disease is second to cancer as a cause of death in both age ranges.

These figures are typical of industrialized countries, but there is some variation. France, noted for its gastronomic excellence, seems to fare better in cardiac matters. Variations in the incidence of the disease occur from region to region within a country. Consequently Eastern Karelia (in Finland) or Scotland have become notorious black spots for coronaries, which makes them centres of clinical research interest.

It may seem a simple matter to identify differences between dietary or other habits from one country to another. Unfortunately geographical, social, genetic and culinary differences are legion and often interdependent, so that a single or simple cause cannot be exposed with certainty. Therefore epidemiology is a very valuable tool in demonstrating possible risk factors, but it cannot prove causality. Sensible use of this information, combined with other evidence from human and animal experiments, can give rise to intelligent theories. It is from here that one can plan some action against the appalling death rates from these diseases and take steps to avoid unnecessary risks.

Fig. 1. Causes of death in men and women aged 45 to 54 years and 35 to 44 years, in England and Wales 1973.

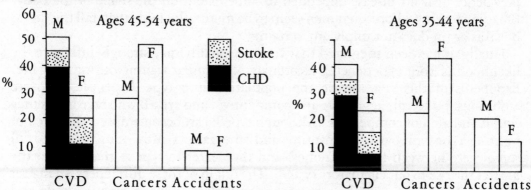

CVD = All Cardiovascular Diseases
CHD = Coronary Heart Disease
M = Male
F = Female

From JOURNAL OF ROYAL COLLEGE OF PHYSICIANS, Vol. 10, No. 3, April 1976.

Unavoidable Risks

There are a number of risk factors which cannot be avoided, and one of these is being male. It is true that some men can and do live to a ripe old age, but others appear to suffer from coronary events with much greater frequency than women and at a much earlier age. It has been suggested that female hormones offer a protection to women, at least in the first part of their lives, but this is not to say that premature death should be regarded as inevitable for men.

Another obvious factor is that of ageing, since with a few exceptions clinical manifestations of arterial disorders become apparent with increasing age. We all know that the tissues of both humans and animals age and ultimately die, although they are continually replaced during life. The process of ageing has fascinated scientists for decades and although various theories have been proposed there is no clear answer available. It is probably true that changes in arteries and blood capillaries occur in all elderly people. However, a disturbance leading to a coronary or a stroke is not an inevitable consequence of ageing, and undoubtedly life could be prolonged if we could avoid such diseases. Women have an average life expectancy five or six years greater than that of men.

There are genetic factors at work which appear to make some families more susceptible than others, and since it is not possible to change the family into which you have been born, this appears to have some importance in heart disease and related disorders. Hard-nosed insurance companies will always ask about diseases in your family, because their experience enables them to assess the risk in accepting you as a client. There are many factors which may precipitate a clinical condition, hence the vulnerability of a family to one particular factor may well be greater or less than that of another family also at risk. If you have relatives who have suffered from these diseases, you should not regard it as inevitable that the same will happen to you, as an elementary study of genetics will demonstrate. Nevertheless, it is perhaps wise to take special care of yourself. In most cases, genetic influences simply render people more or less susceptible to environmental factors which can lead to future problems. It is only in a minority of cases, where detectable inherited disorders of metabolism can be demonstrated, that this is less true.

Another curious result of epidemiological studies was the discovery that the prevalence of heart disease depended to some extent on the shape of the body. Broadly speaking, short squat men seem to be more vulnerable than tall thin ones, but this again does not imply any certainty.

Finally, it has been suggested that your personality may strongly influence the likelihood of your experiencing a coronary or a similar trauma during your life. Exponents of this view divide the population into type A people, who are ambitious, punctual, aggressive and competitive, and type B who take life as they find it and are not competitive. Although type B can become upset, they are not fighting a constant battle against time and other factors. Most of us are said to fall somewhere between these extremes, and the nearer to type A that we are, the greater the risk to our circulatory system. The origin of these differences is a matter of great debate, i.e. whether they are inherited or induced by our family and cultural environment. What is certain is that these behaviour patterns are not easily changed, and that there is little in the organization of industrialized society to relieve us from anxiety. On the contrary, there is every inducement to competition and aggression, either behind the wheel of a motor car or relative to our colleagues at work. Radical self-assessment may enable you to make some changes which could be beneficial not only to your personal happiness but also to your arteries.

Assessing Your Risk

In evaluating the risk of arterial disease in an individual prior to any clinical events, all the above factors should be taken into account. There are additional measurements which can be made to further the assessment.

Blood Fats

It is widely believed in the medical world that a high level of fat circulating in the blood can increase the risk of heart disease, and it can be shown that among people who ultimately suffer a heart attack or stroke, a much higher proportion have raised levels of fat in their blood as compared with the apparently healthy members of a community. It is now possible to analyse blood for fats, using automated techniques, but this process is not normally carried out for individuals without clinical symptoms.

In conversation we think of fats as the common household types such as lard, beef fat, butter or margarine. These are indeed chemically very similar to some of the fats found in the blood and those stored in the body, which biochemists term triglycerides, but there are also other types: the phospholipids and — more notorious and chemically different — cholesterol. These share the property of being very insoluble in water, which is the basic solvent of the blood. Fats are transported in the blood by forming complexes (lipoproteins) with different types of proteins, in much the same way that fat is stabilized in milk. It has now been shown that these lipoproteins are of vital importance in the development of arterial disease.

In general the triglycerides are used as energy reserves and are by far the largest pool of fat: too large in some people (*see* section on obesity below). Phospholipids and cholesterol are essential parts of the structure of cells, the basic units of all human tissues. Cholesterol is found in large amounts in the brain and nervous tissues, and similar quantities are found in people whose dietary cholesterol intake is low since cholesterol can be made from other simple food materials, especially in the liver and intestines. It is only an abnormality in the distribution of these fats which can create problems, and under normal circumstances the cholesterol in your body is not quite the menace that it is sometimes made out to be. Cholesterol forms an essential part of the structure of the thin membranes which surround all the cells in our tissues and organs, and influences the movement of nutrients in and out of cells; it is only when it becomes deposited in large amounts, unassociated with the membranes of arterial cells, that we recognize an abnormality.

Abnormalities of blood fats have been shown to be inherited in a minority of cases where very high blood levels of cholesterol, triglyceride or both can be observed in childhood. In most cases these young people run a very high risk of suffering a coronary in their twenties, thus providing part of the evidence for an association between blood fats and heart disease. The severity of such disorders depends on whether the genes have been inherited from one or both parents, but the majority of blood fat abnormalities cannot so easily be traced to genetic causes, although they may underlie some of them. In many instances they may be secondary to other disorders, but often there is no apparent cause. In a population with no known health problems approximately 15 per cent have high levels of blood fats. In patients with heart disease this is more in the order of 50 per cent, which also indicates that blood fats are not the only factors involved. They cannot, however, be ignored. It may be worth mentioning that it is difficult to define normal levels of blood fats in a population and to say what is abnormal or too high. The 'normal' value for an adult European or North American male is about 2.25 grams per litre of serum, and values above this are considered to be suspect. However, in many African tribes the normal value is below 2.0 grams per litre and in some cases below 1.5. There are some individuals in industrialized countries with cholesterol levels as low as this.

A prospective study of the inhabitants in the town of Framingham, Massachussetts, indicated that people with high blood cholesterol levels were at risk, and this seemed to be especially true for the younger male age group (35 to 45 years).

However, the risk is compounded by the existence of other factors such as cigarette smoking and high blood pressure. Later studies showed that high blood triglyceride levels were also equally prevalent among survivors of heart attacks. For example, a very recent study comparing 40-year-old men in Edinburgh and Stockholm showed that the prevailing blood cholesterol levels were similar in the two cities, despite the fact that the incidence of heart disease is much higher in Edinburgh for men of this age group. However, the blood triglyceride levels of the Scots were higher, but they also smoke more and there were as usual other complicating factors. It is possible to have raised levels of both triglyceride and cholesterol, which is considered to be an even greater risk. High blood triglyceride concentrations may be of greater consequence later in life.

Cigarette Smoking

There is considerable unanimity among research workers that cigarette smoking constitutes a significant risk in coronary heart disease. This has become clear from the Framingham and subsequent studies, which showed that the risk increased with the number of cigarettes smoked. Death from a coronary is uncommon for non-smokers under 45 years of age, whereas the risk for those smoking 40 cigarettes a day can be up to ten times greater than for a non-smoker in the age group 45 to 55. After that age smoking contributes less to the overall risk, which is in any case higher. It should be stressed that there are considerable reductions in risk for smokers who abandon the habit, and that pipe and cigar smoking seems to be less of a problem if the smokers do not inhale.

The main agent in cigarette smoke is likely to be the gas carbon monoxide, which displaces oxygen from the red cells of the blood. This seems to give rise to local arterial damage and increases the tendency of the blood to form a clot or thrombus.

Blood Pressure

Most people have experienced a blood pressure measurement in their doctor's surgery or hospital at some time in their lives. Two measurements are taken since blood pressure changes with the contraction of the heart. Basically a maximum (systolic) and minimum (diastolic) pressure are taken, which ideally should be 120 and 80 mm of mercury respectively. For reasons which are not fully understood, the measurements are higher than this in large sections of the population and there is a relationship between increased diastolic or systolic blood pressure and heart disease. This condition, known as hypertension, may exist for years without any apparent ill effects.

Hypertension does appear to be more prevalent with increasing age, and as a risk factor in heart disease has much greater importance in men of 55 and above and in elderly women. While hypertension can be treated with drugs, it is difficult to prescribe these on a virtually permanent basis unless the case is severe. Nevertheless a study in the United States on middle-aged men showed considerable benefits from this kind of treatment in that the mortality from heart disease was halved.

Mild hypertension is therefore a risk factor in its own right, and it renders the sufferer more susceptible to other risk factors such as smoking and elevated blood fats. It is possible to calculate, for instance, that in the United States the probability of a 35-year-old man with normal blood fats developing coronary heart disease within the next twenty years is approximately 1 in 20, compared with a risk of 1 in 7 for a man of the same age with high blood fat level. The latter ratio can be increased to 1 in 5 for a smoker, and to 1 in 3 if there is also a risk from hypertension. The combination of high blood fats, smoking and hypertension can give a probable risk of over 1 in 2 for men of 45 years and over, and 1 in 6 for women in the same age range. The combined effects of cholesterol, smoking and hypertension are shown in Fig.2, where the mortality over a ten-year period for men aged 30 to 59 has been calculated from a number of separate studies. Over a ten-year period the probability rates are, as one would expect, lower (2 in 100) for a non-smoking normotensive individual with normal blood lipids.

Other Risk Factors

Diabetes

Many people think that all the problems of diabetes have been solved by the discovery of insulin and its clinical application. It is true that many lives have been saved in this way, but diabetics do suffer from various long-term difficulties even when treated. Changes in small blood vessels create problems in the kidneys, eyes and other organs, but there is also an increased risk of coronary heart disease among diabetics as compared with non-diabetics. The main recommendation is even stricter control of other risk factors such as diet, smoking and blood pressure.

Fig. 2. Combined effects of plasma cholesterol, cigarette smoking and hypertension on the risk of CHD. Ten-year rates per 1,000 for first major CHD events in men aged 30 to 59 years at entry. U.S.A. National Cooperative Pooling Project (Stamler and Epstein, 1972).

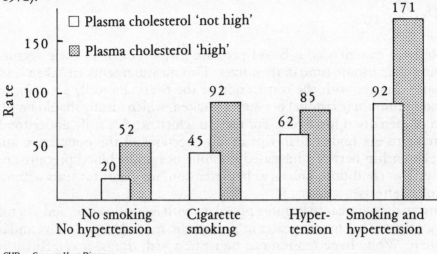

CHD = Coronary Heart Disease

From JOURNAL OF ROYAL COLLEGE OF PHYSICIANS, Vol. 10, No. 3, April 1976.

It is interesting that many people with various forms of arterial disease have a sub-clinical diabetic condition in that, following a test meal of glucose, it takes longer than normal for their blood glucose levels to return to the basal level. This abnormal glucose tolerance is sometimes used, along with other measurements, as an indicator of risk in apparently healthy individuals.

Obesity

It is widely believed by the general public that overweight people are more likely to experience a heart attack. There is ample evidence from the major insurance companies that excess body weight is a bad business risk for them, as is proved by their statistics. This is a broad generalization covering deaths from all causes and does not specify the importance of obesity in arterial disease. While it appears that people who are 20 per cent or more above their ideal weight run an increased risk of coronary heart disease, except in the case of gross overweight this is of lesser importance than the factors mentioned above. In some cases it is associated with high blood triglyceride levels, high blood pressure and glucose intolerance; therefore it is a worthwhile project for an overweight person to shed this excess.

Physical Inactivity

One side of the obesity coin is reduced physical activity, which is again considered by the public to be a crucial factor in relation to heart disease. People are probably conscious of the fact that their lives have become increasingly sedentary, both at work and at home, but only a minority try to rectify this.

Existing evidence on the significance of physical inactivity is not entirely conclusive. A study of London busmen performed some years ago showed that bus conductors were less inclined to coronary disease than their fellow drivers, which indicated that exercise may be important. However, in some agricultural areas such as eastern Finland and the West of Scotland, where there is plenty of heavy work, the incidence of heart disease is also very high, yet within certain industries those workers engaged in heavy work appear to be afforded some protection.

It appears that brisk or vigorous exercise may well be of value. Recent evidence from California, where jogging is a favoured form of exercise, showed that favourable changes in the proportion of different types of blood lipoproteins were noticed in joggers. Exercise like swimming, jogging, rapid walking, cycling or heavy jobs around the house is probably beneficial, but it should not be regarded as a means of counteracting the effects of smoking or other risk factors. There is evidence that exercise will lower blood triglyceride levels, but those who have long forgotten the sensation of exertion should break themselves in gently, since sudden strenuous exercise can also be dangerous in middle age.

Stress

We have already mentioned in the section on unavoidable risks the possibility that personality type may be of importance, and that this is related to the general question of stress and heart disease. There is a considerable division of opinion among medical experts on the significance of stress, some pointing to the transitory effects of stress on blood pressure, blood fats and pulse rate, and others questioning the importance of short-term changes. It has been suggested that general worry may be less important than the stopwatch stress of a busy working life, but this theory does not appear to square with the fact that the incidence of heart disease is very high in some agricultural areas where that kind of stress is unexpected. It could well be argued that in these cases other causal factors are more significant than the absence of stress. Similarly the protection gained by women has been attributed to their less stressful lives, a fact which many women today would hotly dispute. Active and busy lives may involve a certain degree of stress, but can also give enjoyment and be stimulating. There is probably a distinction between hard work and being so overtaxed that symptoms such as depression, sleeplessness and irritability become commonplace in your life, at which point there is clearly a need for change for a number of reasons, apart from the question of heart disease.

Diet

We can now turn our attention to the factor which causes most controversy: that of diet. Earlier in this chapter we mentioned the importance of food in the development of the human race. Dietary habits are something which individuals feel more able to control than cigarette smoking. We should emphasize that eating a prudent diet will not automatically overcome the other risk factors we have already mentioned, e.g. cigarette smoking, and also that individuals are likely to be as sensitive to different dietary factors as they are to various non-dietary ones. Here we have to sift a vast accumulation of information taken from epidemiological studies, and experiments with animals and on human volunteers, which strongly indicates that diet is an important factor in heart disease.

Cholesterol

At the beginning of this century, the Russian scientist Anitschkow fed cholesterol to rabbits and noted pathological changes in their arteries, which in some ways resembled those found in cases of human arterial disease. Later it was found that much of the fatty deposits in diseased arteries also consisted of cholesterol, although small quantities of cholesterol are also found in normal arteries. It was natural to suspect a close association between dietary cholesterol and coronary heart disease, supported by the later discovery that children with inherited high blood cholesterol levels are early victims of heart attacks. A number of everyday foods contain cholesterol (*see* Table 5), especially those of animal origin, and eggs top the list with about 0.3 gram per egg. In the 1950s the main emphasis was placed on dietary cholesterol as a principal cause of elevated blood cholesterol levels and therefore heart disease; so low-cholesterol diets were therefore recommended. In the United States this extended to restaurants preparing low-cholesterol meals and to the cholesterol content of foods being stated on their packaging. While this view is still held, the matter has become more complex because it is now believed that cholesterol itself may not be as important in determining blood cholesterol levels as the type of fat eaten in the diet, although opinions do vary.

Table 5.   Cholesterol Composition of Foods[a]

FOOD	Cholesterol content (mg / 100 g. food) [b]		
Milk, cow's fresh	14	pork	72
skimmed	2	chicken, light meat	69
condensed, whole, sweetened	34	chicken, dark meat	110
Butter	230	duck	110
Cream, single	66	turkey, light meat	49
double	140	turkey, dark meat	81
Cheese, Cheddar	70	brain	2200
Cottage	13	liver (calf)	370
Yogurt, low fat	7	Meat products	
Egg, whole[c]	450	ham	33
white	0	sausage, beef	40
yolk	1260	sausage, pork	47
Fats and oils		Fish	
dripping, beef	60	cod	50
lard	70	plaice	70
margarine	trace	herring	70
suet	74	mackerel	80
vegetable oils	trace	tuna (canned)	65
Meats (raw, lean and fat)		shrimps	200
bacon	57	roe	500
beef	65	Mayonnaise	260
lamb	78		

a   from A.A. Paul and D.A.T. Southgate (1978) **McCance and Widdowson's The Composition of Foods**, Her Majesty's Stationery Office, London.
b   100 g food = approximately 3 ½ oz
c   1 egg = approximately 50 g

Recent evidence on the cholesterol content of Scottish diets shows that they contain no more than those in England, where the incidence of heart disease is lower. On the whole, dietary cholesterol intake is higher in the richer industrialized countries, and epidemiological evidence shows a strong positive correlation between such intake and heart disease. However, the Masai people of Kenya pose an interesting problem to medical scientists, since although they consume large amounts of dairy produce and blood from their herds of cattle and goats, thereby having a similar or higher consumption of cholesterol than people in industrialized countries, they have no clinical manifestations of heart disease and only minor arterial abnormalities. There is some support for the idea that these nomadic people are more able to suppress the synthesis of cholesterol in their own bodies when cholesterol is fed in the diet. Animals such as the rat and dog can do this, but the rabbit does not have the same flexibility. Experiments on human volunteers in the United States and other countries indicate that this response to cholesterol in the diet does exist, but not as effectively as in the Masai. So many other things are different about the life of a nomadic tribesman, that it is difficult to be certain whether this is a genetic peculiarity of the Masai or a consequence of environmental factors which affect cholesterol balance.

Unfortunately many of the foods which contain cholesterol seem to have other desirable attributes. Eggs, meat, cheese and milk are valuable sources of protein, and unless a strict low-cholesterol diet has been advised by a clinician it is not intended that these be cut out. Poultry and fish are suggested as alternatives because of their lower fat content (*see* below). A rule of thumb on eggs for healthy individuals is about three a week. Where low-cholesterol diets have been specifically advised this will mean avoidance of egg yolks, liver, kidney and a lower consumption of all animal products.

Fat

Fats contribute a great deal to our diet, not only as one of the main components of the total intake, but also as to the palatability of our food. Low-fat diets consumed in Third World countries often seem boring or less satisfying than those containing at least a moderate amount of fat. Nutritionists have noted that the total contribution of fats to the number of our food calories has been slowly rising and is now approximately 42 per cent in northern Europe and America. Some years ago Ancel Keys, an American nutritionist, found a positive correlation between the total fat consumption in a number of countries and the incidence of heart disease. This relationship was shown to be even closer when the consumption of fats from animal sources was studied, with the United States, United Kingdom and Scandinavian countries near the top of the list. There was evidence from experimental animals such as rabbits and cockerels that those fed diets rich in animal fats developed more fatty degeneration of the arteries than those eating plant oils. Included in the animal fats are butter, lard and beef fat.

In their basic chemical structure, animal fats and plant oils are very similar, but obviously they have very different physical properties in that the fats are solid and the oils liquid. Hard fats consist primarily of carbon atoms linked to each other in chains or to atoms of hydrogen (not too dissimilar to the hydrocarbons of gasoline, but longer chains). These chains pack tightly alongside each other and because of this, readily solidify. In oils the carbon chains do not have their full complement of hydrogen atoms and are said to be unsaturated with hydrogen compared with the saturated solid fats. This lack of hydrogen gives rise to bends in the normally straight chains, and prevents the close packing seen in solid fats. Therefore we experience these unsaturated fats as liquid oils, such as olive oil or peanut oil, simply because they are more disorganized. Some oils have more than one point of unsaturation along their carbon chains and are termed polyunsaturates, examples being corn and sunflower oils.

Oils and fats have three carbon chains for each molecule, and can consist of a mixture of saturated, unsaturated and polyunsaturated chains which are chemically linked. An important point to remember is that animals can make saturated and unsaturated fats from other food constituents, but some polyunsaturates — especially those containing the carbon chain of linoleic acid — cannot be thus made and have to be obtained from plant sources or from the lean meat of animals which eat plants.

Having gone to some lengths to understand fats and oils we should return to their use in human nutrition. Butter and animal fats have formed part of our diet for centuries, but alternatives — such as the introduction of margarine — have been produced by manufacturers in response to the demands of military food requirements. In their normal state, oils are unacceptable for spreading on bread, therefore a process was invented to saturate whale and vegetable oils with hydrogen and render them solid. By the use of colouring agents and careful blending, the product is fairly close in texture and flavour to butter. Other products can resemble a hard cooking fat like lard. Thus margarine and vegetable cooking fats have partially replaced butter and lard in the modern shopping basket.

Experimentation has shown that feeding polyunsaturates to human volunteers reduced the level of blood fats, especially cholesterol. Butter contains only 2 per cent of polyunsaturates and the margarines somewhat more (Table 6). New margarines are now widely available, albeit more expensive, which contain large amounts of polyunsaturates but by technological cunning are made sufficiently solid for the required spreading properties. These margarines are also advertised as cholesterol-free. The possibility therefore exists for you to pick the type of fat you wish to consume. Vegetable oils have always been available and most vegetables contain polyunsaturates, although the total fat content is usually low in most vegetables.

The big question is, 'How much will an increase in the dietary polyunsaturates protect a population against coronary heart disease?' This is always a difficult point to prove conclusively in a lifelong degenerative disease, because no one will volunteer for experiments for that time! Nevertheless a number of dietary intervention studies have been carried out in the United States and Finland. In the latter case inmates of two mental institutions were involved, and were given either a diet with the normal saturated fat of Finnish food or a modified diet in which large portions of the fat were polyunsaturated, including margarine and skimmed milk 'filled' with soya bean oil. The investigators found that this substitution brought about a reduction in the number of deaths from heart disease over the years, but other studies have been less successful in producing clear-cut results.

There is little information on the effects of lifelong consumption of large

Table 6.   Fatty Acid Composition of Foods [a]

FOOD	FATTY ACIDS (g / 100 g total fatty acids)		
	Saturated	Mono-unsaturated	Polyunsaturated
Flour (wholemeal & white)	20.2	16.2	63.7
Baked beans	21.3	12.1	63.0
Potatoes	23.2	3.2	73.7
Fancy iced cakes	65.6	27.8	5.8
Milk (cows') and butter	61.1	31.9	2.9
Eggs	37.9	47.1	11.1
Fats and oils			
dripping, beef	43.1	48.3	4.3
lard	44.0	44.0	9.5
hard margarine			
animal & veg. oils	37.5	44.7	16.0
veg. oils only	38.2	48.9	12.6
soft margarine			
animal & veg. oils	30.7	47.1	20.4
veg. oils only	33.1	43.5	23.1
polyunsaturated marg			
veg. oil only	24.7	20.5	54.6
suet	57.7	36.5	1.3
vegetable oils			
coconut	75.9	7.0	1.8
cottonseed	26.8	22.3	50.4
maize (corn)	17.2	30.7	51.6
olive	14.7	73.0	11.7
palm	47.4	43.6	8.7
peanut, groundnut	19.7	50.1	29.8
safflower seed	10.7	13.2	75.5
soya bean	14.7	25.4	59.4
sunflower seed	13.7	33.3	52.3
Meats			
bacon	43.3	47.9	7.8
beef	44.9	49.3	4.3
lamb	52.1	40.5	5.0
pork	42.5	47.9	8.3
chicken	35.1	47.6	14.9
duck	28.9	57.2	12.7
liver, calf	41.2	23.4	31.8
ham	39.2	48.8	10.4
sausage, beef	44.4	49.1	5.0
sausage, pork	41.3	49.5	8.3
steak & kidney pie	42.8	41.9	10.9
Fish			
cod	26.1	15.9	56.8
plaice	23.4	38.5	33.7
herring	22.3	55.8	19.6
mackerel	27.0	41.3	27.1
tuna (canned)	18.8	41.0	38.3
Nuts			
almonds	8.3	71.6	19.6
coconut	83.0	7.0	1.8
peanuts	15.2	50.1	29.8

[a]   calculated from data A.A. Paul and D.A.T. Southgate (1978) **McCance and Widdowson's The Composition of Foods**, Her Majesty's Stationery Office, London.

amounts of polyunsaturates, and it has been suggested that this may increase the dietary requirements for vitamin E, which protects polyunsaturates from rancidity as a result of contact with oxygen. In terms of our total fat intake it is recommended that this should be reduced from 42 per cent of the total calories to 35 per cent, i.e. spreading your margarine more thinly, eating lean meat (especially poultry and some fish) and grilling rather than frying in fat. It is also suggested that a greater proportion of this fat should be in the form of polyunsaturates, but this does not mean a wholesale rejection of all saturated fat-containing foods. Milk, for instance, is a valuable food especially for children. Experiments have shown that there is a substance in milk which reduces the amount of cholesterol made by the body and that yogurt has blood cholesterol-lowering properties. Low-fat varieties of dairy products are commonly available and these should be bought where possible. It should be emphasized that fresh vegetables and salads will also increase the dietary intake of polyunsaturates. Again, lean meats, poultry and fish will increase the proportion of polyunsaturates to saturated fats. More sparing use of butter is desirable, with the substitution of polyunsaturated margarines but not ordinary margarines.

These indictments against saturated fats have had a profound effect on the dairy industry. In Australia there has been some success in producing a 'polyunsaturated cow' to increase the linoleic acid content of their milk and beef. Most dietary fats are hydrogenated in the rumen of the cow and the milk contains little polyunsaturated fat. There is a limit to the extent to which people will reduce favoured and often valuable foods, unless there is an immediate medical reason for doing so. A sensible compromise can be reached by partially substituting polyunsaturates from other sources.

Polyunsaturates are used in combination with cholesterol-lowering drugs in the treatment of definable genetic disorders, where blood cholesterol levels are very high. Polyunsaturate-rich diets are also advised for people with high blood cholesterol levels of indeterminate origin, in combination with a low cholesterol diet (see previous section). There is some disagreement on the mode of action of polyunsaturates in the body. It is variously suggested that they reduce the absorption of cholesterol, increase its excretion, decrease its synthesis or move cholesterol from the blood into the tissues. Having stated earlier that polyunsaturates are essential to our diet, it is more difficult to say that populations which are susceptible to heart disease are actually deficient in polyunsaturated fats, in the sense of a vitamin deficiency. However, there seems to be a strong case for a reduction in the total intake of all fats and a bigger proportion of polyunsaturates in the remainder.

Sugar

One of the most remarkable changes in our diet since the Industrial Revolution has been the inclusion of purified cane sugar which now, on average, contributes up to 20 per cent of our total calorie intake. This figure may be higher in the case of children and a few adults. Up to 450 grams a day was recorded in some Iowa school-children, and in surveys of lunch-time habits in England, individual children with sugar intakes of up to 50 per cent of total calories were discovered. This change has been largely at the expense of starchy foods, particularly bread, which together with sugar form the main carbohydrate components of our diet. The contribution of carbohydrate to our total energy intake is around 45 per cent. The main reason for this transformation was the invention of industrial processes which reduced the price of cane sugar and brought it within the reach of all the population, who were attracted by its obvious palatability. Other sugars like glucose and fructose contribute only a small amount to the modern diet, although this is increasing with the development of processes which can make these sugars cheaply from corn starch. Artificial sweeteners have been replacing sugar in some food products, but have come under attack as cancer-producing agents.

For a long time it was thought that one carbohydrate was metabolized in the body much like another, but this is now known to be not exactly true. An epidemiological study by Professor John Yudkin showed that there was an equally strong relationship between the incidence of coronary heart diseases in a series of countries and their consumption of sugar, as there is with their animal fat consumption. In the case of both dietary constituents, it is difficult to prove that consumption of fat or sugar for particular individuals makes them more susceptible to heart disease. No large-scale diet intervention studies have been attempted with sugar as there have been with dietary fat, hence we have to look for indirect evidence.

A favourite device of epidemiologists is to study populations which have migrated from one country to another and adopted different food habits. Jews emigrating from the Yemen were found to have more diabetes and heart disease after a period in Israel and this was attributed mainly to their increased sugar consumption. Eskimos who have forsaken their traditional diets rich in protein and fat and now consume the usual North American fare (including large amounts of sugar), exhibit abnormalities of glucose body chemistry reminiscent of pre-diabetes states. Other scientists, however, point to sugar cane cutters, who eat large amounts of cane at various times of the year but do not suffer from coronary heart disease. However, this sugar has not been refined.

Experiments with animals and humans have shown that increased sugar intake increases blood triglyceride levels, although in humans these effects may be transitory. It should be remembered that in human studies the volunteers usually have a previous dietary history of sugar consumption, and it has been demonstrated in animal experiments that the feeding of young animals with sugar can leave a permanent imprint. This means that triglyceride levels may stay high even when the animals are transferred from a sugar diet to a starchy diet when grown, compared with the lower triglyceride levels found in animals which have eaten the starch diets since birth (weaning). Animal and human experiments also indicate that exercise can override the triglyceride-raising effects of sugar. Individuals moreover respond differently to sugar: some, more sensitive than others, may have raised triglyceride or even insulin concentration in their blood.

Experiments with animals showing arterial disease as a result of sugar feeding have been less successful, but further work is needed on more suitable animal models. It is possible to produce changes in the small blood vessels of experimental animals, which are similar to those produced in experimental and human diabetes affecting the kidneys and the eyes.

Apart from its contribution to our already large energy consumption, sugar has no other nutrients because it is so highly purified and is in no way essential in our diet (brown sugar is also highly purified). A small amount of carbohydrate is necessary in our diet, but this can be supplied as starch. A reduction in sugar intake is of value in obesity and may therefore reduce the risk of a coronary, but one problem is that so many food products include sugar. Less than half of our consumption is directly added by the consumer and we are therefore usually unaware of the total amount of sugar we are consuming.

Fibre

Sugars and starches are the main components of dietary carbohydrates but there are some indigestible carbohydrates (fibre) which are present in small amounts especially in foods of plant origin (*see* Chapter I). It has been suggested that the low level of dietary fibre contributes to the high incidence of coronary heart disease. One of the major routes for losing cholesterol and its breakdown products, bile salts, from the body is through the bowel. It is thought by some that dietary fibre may promote this loss and reduce blood cholesterol levels. The chemical composition of fibre varies from one source to another and although fibre in wholemeal bread receives the greatest publicity there is no certainty that it produces the best effects. White bread is often severely criticized, sometimes unfairly, because it still contains valuable nutrients especially in comparison with other foods. There is no disadvantage in increasing fibre in the diet by increasing the consumption of wholemeal bread at the expense of non-sugary food, and also by eating more vegetables and fruit. From an overall nutritional standpoint this will be of great value and a positive advantage from the standpoint of coronary heart disease and other disorders.

Vitamins

In some circles, there is a popular belief that our main dietary problem is a shortage of vitamins, a view which conventional professional opinion does not support. Vitamin C, which has gained a reputation for itself as a cure-all in other spheres, has been implicated in the development of heart disease. It has been suggested that vitamin C lowers blood fat concentration, but the results of a variety of experiments have been contradictory and on balance the weight of the evidence is against such effects.

Excess vitamin D intake has also been suggested as a factor in heart disease. Over-zealous feeding of this vitamin to the young can give rise to problems, including calcification of tissues which does also occur in diseased arteries. In the north of Norway, where vitamin D is consumed in large amounts in fish livers, it is claimed that calcification of kidney tissues is related to the occurrence of heart disease.

Minerals and Water Hardness

The view has been expressed that some minerals such as magnesium have a protective action against coronaries. Magnesium is found in many foods, especially green vegetables and milk. There have been suggestions that the amount of magnesium in our diet is sometimes marginally less than the recommended level, whereas at one time dietary magnesium was thought to be more than adequate. Alcohol and other food substances can enhance the excretion of magnesium in urine. Low magnesium consumption may increase the blood cholesterol levels, but as yet the evidence is inconclusive. Other research workers maintain that the lack of certain trace elements like chromium may be of central importance, and have some interesting experimental evidence to support their views.

One of the surprising epidemiological findings of the last few years was that the incidence of coronaries in areas where the water is soft (low in minerals) is greater than in those where mineral-rich hard water is supplied because of the geographical location. It has been hard to pin down a cause, but it may well be connected with the dissolved minerals, mainly calcium and magnesium, although these contribute only a small proportion of our dietary requirements. The main recommendation must be that eating a nutritious and varied diet which includes plenty of fresh fruit and green vegetables will eliminate the possibility of any dietary lack of minerals.

You may have noticed that there has so far been no suggestion of a connection between diet and high blood pressure (although there is some slight evidence that high sugar intakes may increase blood pressure). The best known mineral is of course common salt, and it has been proposed that the high salt intake in industrialized countries is responsible for the prevalence of hypertension. In the United Kingdom there is currently a national survey on the prevalence of hypertension in the community. There has been no attempt to show that reducing salts in the diet has any effect on coronary heart disease, but it may well be a good idea to cut down on salt consumption, especially in view of the fact that salt is already present in many manufactured foods and even in frozen vegetables.

Alcohol and Coffee

The serious effects of excess alcohol drinking are well known. There is, however, little direct evidence that alcohol is harmful in relation to heart disease. There is a tendency for alcohol, even in moderate amounts, to increase blood triglyceride concentration, and it can also contribute to problems of overweight since it is a rich source of calories.

Since most pleasures become suspect, the habit of coffee drinking was scrutinized and it was found that more coffee was drunk by people who had suffered coronaries than by their healthy counterparts. Others have suggested that this association is due to the fact that smokers tend to drink more coffee and frequently this also means an increase in sugar intake. Coffee itself appears not to be a serious risk factor on the existing evidence.

Current Trends

Medical statisticians have anxiously watched the inexorable rise in deaths from heart disease over the last few decades and have noticed how younger people, especially men, were becoming increasingly vulnerable. Autopsies on young soldiers who fell in the Korean and Vietnam wars revealed that at 18 to 20 years of age, the major arteries were severely affected in some individuals. It was first noticed in the United States, where public information on these problems was more widely disseminated, that this increased mortality levelled off and there is now a small but definite decline. Very recent figures from the United Kingdom have also shown this encouraging trend among men. Epidemiologists have naturally been concerned to account for the cause of this improvement, however small. There has been a significant decline in cigarette smoking, especially among the professional classes. In the United Kingdom and United States there has been a movement towards the increased consumption of polyunsaturated fats at the expense of animal fats such as lard. In the UK the use of butter or margarine has fluctuated according to their relative prices. The use of vegetable and salad oil increased, but the consumption of total fats declined slightly. Total liquid milk and cream consumption showed no clear changes over the last eight years and the number of eggs consumed per person per week declined over the same period by about half an egg to four eggs per person per week. The largest percentage change in any food was a reduction in refined and icing sugar consumption by about one-third, but this did not take account of the disguised sugar in manufactured foods. Similar trends in sugar consumption have been recorded in the United States.

Obviously one cannot select one particular factor as crucial, but this is perhaps less important if the exhortations of experts and general practitioners have had some impact on the public. It is likely that this advice is not reaching all strata of society and that wider educational services would improve matters even further. One can only hope that the trend will continue.

In the next chapter the main conclusions of the section on diet will be summarized. On the non-dietary side, we can recommend giving up cigarette smoking, taking consistent exercise and not allowing your life to be regulated by the clock. These are especially effective if you are male and if you have a family history of this disease. You will also discover in the following pages that you can enjoy your food as much and even better than before and at the same time safeguard your health.

Introduction to the Recipes

The only way to really know what you are eating is to cook your own food and bake your own bread. For example, if you check the list of ingredients on a package of ice cream, you will often find that it contains vegetable oils. This sounds reassuring, but actually says nothing; quite often coconut oil is used, an unsuitable fat from a cholesterol point of view.

It is important to be a critical consumer. A good rule of thumb is to choose products which have been processed as little as possible, for example brown rice, or wholewheat flour. In general, unprocessed foodstuffs retain more nutritional value than the processed types.

Never buy products without a detailed list of ingredients. A packaged food producer who knows that his product contains only first-class ingredients should have no reason not to declare them.

It can be difficult to change your diet suddenly, whether the decision stems from an increased awareness of the importance of a good diet or whether your doctor has informed you that your cholesterol level is too high and that you should therefore change your eating habits.

The aim of this book is to support and stimulate those who have already decided to change their diet, and also to tempt those who doubt whether this type of food has any excitement to offer the palate. In creating these recipes we have endeavoured to reduce a) the total amount of fat in the diet, b) the amount of saturated fats, balancing with polyunsaturated fats, c) the amount of dietary cholesterol, and d) the consumption of sugar. The recipes are designed to inspire the reader to experiment, and were composed on the assumption that he or she already has a basic knowledge of cooking.

The recipes are for four persons unless otherwise stated.

In the bread recipes we have used fresh yeast as this gives better results. If, however, this is difficult to obtain, a corresponding amount of dried yeast may be used with satisfactory results.

The following is a list of points to keep in mind when choosing or preparing produce. The higher your cholesterol level, the more carefully you should follow these recommendations.

Meat

Choose meat which is as lean as possible. Recommended cuts are:
Beef: Thick flank, fillet steak, rump steak and sirloin.
Pork: Chops, tenderloin and ham.
Lamb: Chops, leg and best end of neck.
Veal: Escalope, neck, fillet of veal and chops.

Limit your intake of offal such as liver, kidney and brains. If the meat is to be boiled it should be boneless as the marrow is rich in saturated fats.

Remove all visible fat from the meat before cooking.

Do not buy ready-minced meat, as even pure minced beef contains too much fat. If you have a friendly butcher, you can ask him to grind the meat for you after he has removed all visible fat; otherwise, grind it yourself.

Try to reduce the amount of meat in your diet. Eat more fish, vegetables, beans and grain foods.

Fowl

Chicken and turkey are suitable birds but goose and duck should be avoided as their flesh contains too much fat.

Remove the skin from the bird before eating, since this contains much saturated fat.

Fish and Shellfish

All types of fish are recommended, even the so-called oily fish as they contain a high percentage of polyunsaturated fats. Fish roes should not be eaten.

Regarding shellfish, the tail and claw meat of shrimps, crayfish, lobster etc. may be eaten, but the roe and heads should be avoided. Oysters, clams, mussels and so on should only be eaten on rare occasions.

Other foodstuffs

Include a variety of fresh fruit and vegetables in your daily diet for valuable vitamins, minerals, some polyunsaturated fats and fibre.

Fresh milk and milk products such as cheese and yogurt should not be discouraged, but where possible low-fat varieties should be used.

Fruit is a far better way of satisfying your sweet tooth than cakes, sweets and sugary cereals.

Try to reduce the amount of sugar which you put in your tea and coffee.

Increase the fibre content of your diet with wholemeal bread and plenty of vegetables and salad.

Healthy individuals can eat about three eggs per week, but where low-cholesterol diets have been advised eggs should be avoided.

Preparation

It is also important to choose the right cooking method: grilling and baking are preferable to frying. When baking meat, place it on a grid over a pan when possible. Do not use the gravy from baked meat, either on its own or as a base for sauces.

When frying always use the recommended oils (see pp. 43) as sparingly as possible. Pour the oil into a cold frying pan and fry your food on a low heat, as you will then need less oil. It is important to remember that polyunsaturated fats are destroyed at high temperatures.

Never deep-fat fry!

A good way to reduce the amount of fat in soups and stews is to let them cool. The fat floats up to the surface, hardens and can then easily be removed before reheating.

We hope that this book will be a practical guide and aid you in changing your diet, and that with its help you will enjoy many delightful, delicious and healthy meals.

Table of Foodstuff Recommendations

In order to make it easier for you to see which foodstuffs are recommended and which are less suitable, we have drawn up a table where the most common and important foodstuffs can easily be found.

In the column to the left you will find foodstuffs which are generally recommended.

In the middle column are listed those foodstuffs with which you should be more careful, particularly if your blood fat level is already too high.

In the column to the right are the foodstuffs with which everyone should be very restrictive.

	RECOMMENDED	USE IN MODERATION	RESTRICT
Vegetables and legumes (pulses)	All fresh veg., potatoes, root veg. beans, lentils mushrooms etc.		Chips Crisps Deep-fat fried onion-rings and other deep-fat fried veg. Tinned, stewed veg. and similar products, containing butter or cream
Fruits and berries	All fresh fruits and berries	Tinned fruit and berries in light syrup Homemade jams, jellies etc. with a min. amount of sugar	Sweetened squash, jam, marmalade, jelly etc. Tinned fruit and berries in heavy syrup
Bread and cereal	Unsweetened bread, preferably wholemeal Crispbread Unsweetened biscuits without filling All cereals such as flour, grains, rice (preferably brown), macaroni, spaghetti etc. Porridge, breakfast cereals etc. without coconut fat, sugar or honey	Homemade cakes and pastries made with polyunsaturated oil or margarine and with a min. amount of sugar Egg noodles	Sweetened bread, cakes cookies, pastries etc.
Dairy products	Low-fat milks such as skimmed milk Low-fat natural yogurt Low-fat cottage cheese	Whole milk Evaporated milk Natural yogurt and sweetened yogurt Cottage cheese Other cheeses	Sweetened, condensed milk Cream, single and double Sour cream Ice cream
Fats	Margarines containing high percentage of polyunsaturated fats Sunflower seed oil Corn oil Soya oil Safflower seed oil Poppy seed oil Cotton seed oil	Olive oil	Butter Other margarines Coconut fat Lard Suet Palm oil
Eggs	Egg white (does *not* contain cholesterol)	3 egg yolks (incl. eggs in manufactured products) per week for those without too high a cholesterol level. Others should try to avoid egg yolks	
Fish and shell-fish	All fish, even the oily types Fish products such as pickled herring, sardines and tuna fish	The tails and claws of prawns, crayfish and lobster	Fish roe Caviar Crab Oyster Deep-fat fried fish
Fowl	Chicken Turkey Wild fowl		Goose Duck

	RECOMMENDED	USE IN MODERATION	RESTRICT
Meat	Veal Game	Lean beef Pork Lamb	Processed meats Bacon Organ meats, e.g. liver, kidneys, brains, sweetbreads Black pudding
Miscellaneous		Sugar and honey (very sparingly) Sorbet	Sweets Chocolate Soft drinks Other products containing much sugar
	All spices Mustard Tomato ketchup Gelatin Bouillon cubes	Salt	
	Mineral water	Beer, wine, sherry, brandy etc. used in cooking and consumed in small quantities	
	Walnuts Almonds Brazil nuts Wheat germ Bran Lin seeds Sesame seeds Poppy seeds	Hazel nuts Peanuts	Coconut Cashews
			All other products containing a large quantity of sugar, eggs and/or saturated fat

Soups

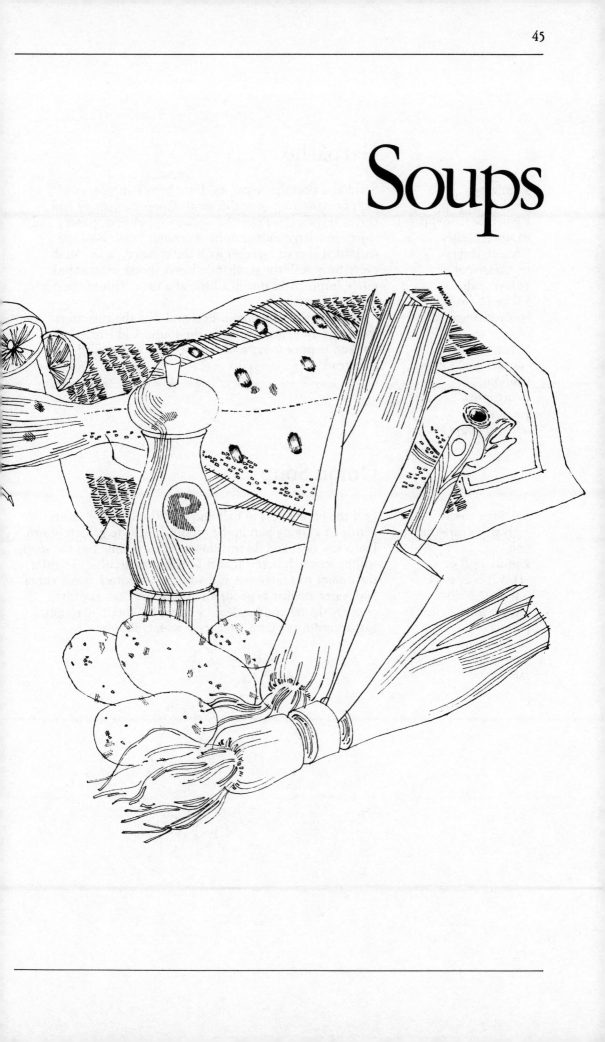

Gazpacho

3 tomatoes
1 red sweet pepper
1 green sweet pepper
1 bunch parsley
1 bunch chives
½ tsp chervil
1 clove garlic
5 fl oz (1.4 dl)
  polyunsaturated
  oil
5 fl oz (1.4 dl)
  water
1 onion
1 cucumber
1 lemon
salt and pepper

Scald and peel the tomatoes. Dice both tomatoes and peppers after removing the seeds. Chop the parsley and chives very finely. Place the tomatoes, peppers, parsley and chives in a large mortar or hard ceramic bowl. Add the crumbled chervil together with the crushed garlic. Mash everything with the pestle or a heavy spoon until a thick purée forms. Add the oil a little at a time. Dilute the purée with cold water.

Peel and slice the onion. Peel and dice the cucumber. Stir the onion and cucumber into the soup. Add lemon juice, salt and pepper to taste. Serve the soup well chilled, with rye bread.

Onion Soup

5-6 large onions
3 tbsp polyunsaturated
  oil
2 pints 13 fl oz
  (1.5 l) beef stock
6 fl oz (1.7 dl)
  white wine
pepper
½ tsp thyme
1 bay leaf
salt

Peel the onions, cut in half and slice thinly. Cook them gently in a frying pan in the oil until they are golden brown. Use a low heat and do this slowly. It takes time but the soup will be so much better that it is worth the trouble. Transfer the onions to a large pot and add the beef stock (stock cubes and water are just as good) and the wine. Season with pepper, thyme and bay leaf. Simmer for about 30 minutes. Salt according to taste, and serve with croûtons.

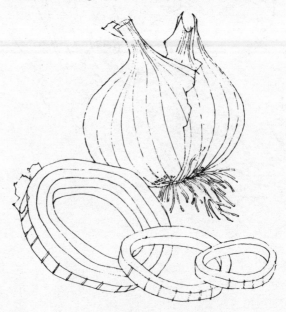

Garlic Soup

12 cloves garlic
4 ripe tomatoes
1 tbsp polyunsaturated
  oil
2 tsp paprika
  powder
2 ¼ pints (1.3 l)
  beef stock
salt and pepper
4 slices toast
parsley

Peel and slice the garlic. Peel and chop the tomatoes. Sauté
the garlic in a saucepan in a little oil for about 2-3 minutes.
Add the tomatoes and allow them to become thoroughly
hot. Dust with the paprika powder and add the beef stock.
Add salt and pepper to taste, then cover and simmer for
about 45 minutes. Place a toasted slice of bread in each soup
bowl and pour on the soup. Sprinkle with parsley and serve.

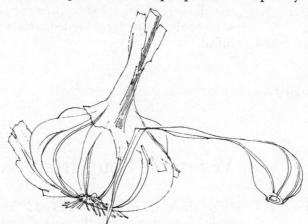

Carrot Soup

8 large carrots
2 pints 2 fl oz (1.2 l)
  beef stock
salt and pepper
parsley

Peel the carrots and grate them coarsely. (Winter carrots are
preferable if obtainable.) Simmer the carrots in a good beef
stock for about 20 minutes. Add salt and pepper about 5
minutes before the end of the cooking time. Sprinkle the
chopped parsley over and serve steaming hot.

Green Pea Soup

6-8 PERSONS

1 lb (454 g) dried green
  peas
4 ½ pints (2.5 l) water
2 carrots
2 potatoes
2-3 onions
2 parsnips
2 ½ tsp salt
black pepper
1 bay leaf
1 tsp marjoram
½ -1 tsp savory

Soak the peas overnight and strain. Put soaked peas in a
saucepan and add 4 ½ pints fresh water. Slice the carrots,
potatoes, onions and parsnips thinly and add to the pan
together with the salt, pepper and bay leaf. Boil for about 2
hours or until the peas can be easily mashed. Press the peas,
onions and other vegetables through a strainer into a second
pan. Add the liquid used to boil the peas and vegetables,
and season with the marjoram and savory.

This recipe yields about 4 ½ pints of soup. As it takes
quite some time to prepare, it is worthwhile making a large
amount and freezing part of it. This soup is suitable both as
a main dish and first course.

Provençal Bean Soup

1 lb (454 g) haricots
  verts
4 potatoes
5-6 ripe tomatoes
1 ¾ pints (1 l) water
  or stock
salt
7 tbsp soup pasta
2 cloves garlic
1 tbsp polyunsaturated
  oil
2 tsp sweet basil
1 tbsp concentrated
  tomato purée
parsley

Rinse, clean and cut the beans into small pieces. Peel the
potatoes and cut them into thin slices. Scald, peel and dice
the tomatoes. Place potatoes and tomatoes in a large
saucepan. Pour on the water or stock, add the salt, and boil
slowly for 20 minutes. Add the beans and pasta, and boil
for a further 10 minutes. (Check the cooking time on the
pasta packet just to make sure.) Mix the crushed garlic with
the oil, sweet basil, tomato purée and chopped parsley, and
stir into the soup. Serve immediately with home-made
bread.

Vegetable Soup from Normandy

1 ¾ pints (1 l) water
2 tsp salt
4 potatoes
2 leeks
8 oz (226 g) haricots
  verts
2 stalks celery
1 small bunch parsley
1 tbsp high-
  polyunsaturated
  margarine
pepper

Bring the water to the boil and add the salt. Add the peeled
and sliced potatoes and the washed and shredded leeks,
then boil for 30 minutes. Cut the haricots verts and celery
into short pieces, and chop the parsley. Add these to the
soup, together with the margarine. Boil the soup until the
haricots verts are soft, about 10 minutes. Add pepper to
taste before serving.

Jerusalem Artichoke Potage

2 lb (9 hg) Jerusalem
  artichokes
1-2 carrots
¾ pint (4.2 dl) water
1 tsp salt
pepper
¾-1 pint (about 5 dl)
  skimmed milk
1 tbsp high-
  polyunsaturated
  margarine
¼ tsp marjoram

Peel the Jerusalem artichokes and carrots, and cut them into
smaller pieces. Place in a large saucepan, add the water, salt
and pepper, cover and boil until the vegetables are soft.
Purée the boiled vegetables in a blender, or press them
through a sieve. Return the purée to the saucepan and add
the skimmed milk to obtain the required soup consistency.
Add the margarine and season with the marjoram and more
salt and pepper if necessary.

Asparagus Soup à la Bertheaud

3-4 medium-sized
  potatoes
1 8-oz (226-g) can
  asparagus
10 fl oz skimmed milk
½ 12-oz (340-g) can
  sweet corn
¼ tsp sweet basil
salt and pepper

Peel, cut up and boil the potatoes in salted water until soft. Drain, and mash the potatoes with the juice from the can of asparagus until smooth. Add the milk and place on a low heat. Stir in the asparagus, corn and basil. Salt and pepper to taste, bring to the boil and serve immediately.

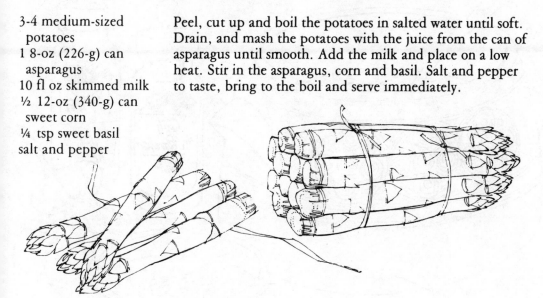

Lentil Soup

2 onions
9 oz (255 g) green
  lentils
2 pints 4 fl oz (1.25 l)
  water
1 bay leaf
salt and pepper

Peel and chop the onions, and place in a saucepan. Add all the other ingredients. Bring to the boil and simmer for about 45 minutes or until the lentils are quite tender and soft.

Goulash Soup

1 lb (454 g) lean beef
2 onions
4 potatoes
1-2 red sweet peppers
1 small carrot
1 14-oz (397-g) can
  tomatoes
1¾ pints (1 l) water
1 stock cube
2 cloves garlic
1 bay leaf
1-1½ tbsp paprika
  powder
1-2 tsp chili powder
salt and pepper

Cut the meat into ½-inch cubes after removing all visible fat. Chop the onion, potatoes, sweet peppers and carrot. Place meat and vegetables in a large saucepan. Add the tomatoes, water, stock cube, crushed garlic, bay leaf, spices and a seasoning of salt and pepper.

Cover the pan and let the soup boil slowly for about 2 hours. Serve with home-made rye bread.

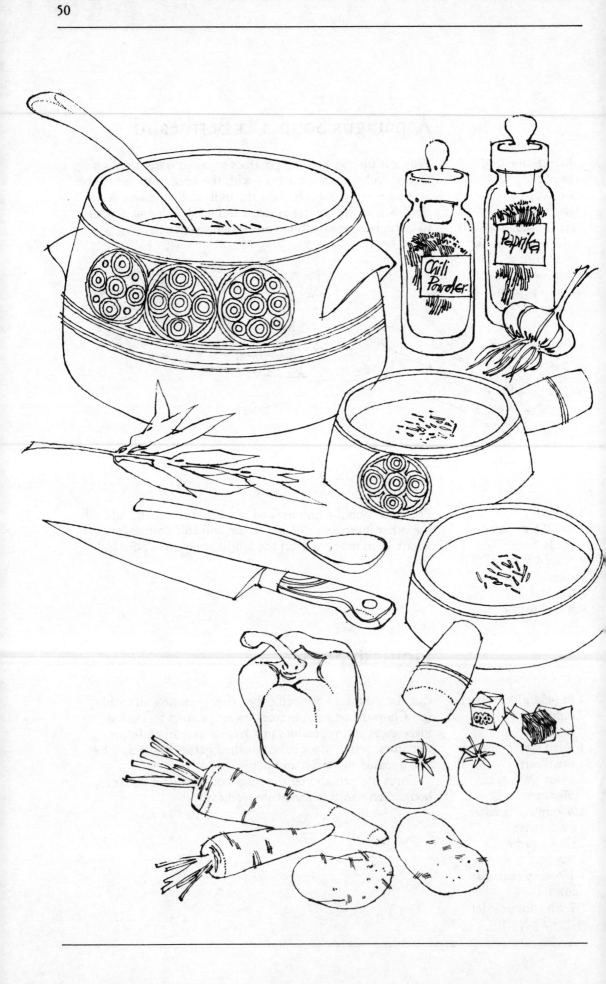

French Fish Soup

about 3 lb (1.4 kg)
  fish, of at least 3
  different kinds
2 onions
2 cloves garlic
1 14-oz (397-g) can
  tomatoes or 6 fresh
  tomatoes
1 bunch parsley
1 head fennel
3 tbsp polyunsaturated
  oil
1 packet saffron
a piece dried orange
  peel
salt and pepper
3½ fl oz (1 dl) white
  wine
8 oz (226 g) prawns
4 crayfish tails

Choose both white and oily fish, for example whiting,
mackerel and plaice. Clean and cut into large pieces.

Peel and chop the onion and garlic, chop the tomatoes,
parsley and fennel; place in a large saucepan together with a
little oil and sauté for a minute or two. Add the spices and
peel, pour on the wine and allow to simmer for a while.

Put in the more compact fish (those that take longer to
cook), and add water to barely cover them. Boil for 7-8
minutes. Add the rest of the fish and boil for a further
7-8 minutes. Add more water if needed.

Add the prawns and crayfish tails just before the soup is
ready. (Do not boil the shellfish tails.) Serve the soup piping
hot with home-made bread.

Hotch-potch

1 lb (454 g) lean
  boneless lamb
3 onions
1½ tbsp high-
  polyunsaturated
  margarine
salt and pepper
2 tbsp pearl barley
2 tsp flour
2 pints 13 fl oz (1.5 l)
  beef stock
2 leeks
2 carrots
1 small cauliflower
1 8-oz (226-g) packet
  frozen peas

Trim away all fat and dice the meat. Peel and chop two of
the onions. Brown the meat cubes with half the chopped
onions in a thick-bottomed saucepan. Add salt and pepper.
When the meat is nicely browned, add the rest of the
chopped onion and the pearl barley. Sprinkle over the flour,
stir and add 7 fl oz (2 dl) of the beef stock. Cover and
simmer until the stock has almost boiled away and the meat
is tender, about 40 minutes. Add more stock if needed.

While the meat is cooking, peel and slice the remaining
onion, the carrots and leeks. Boil these in the rest of the
beef stock for about 20-30 minutes.

About 10 minutes before the end of cooking time, add
the cauliflower, broken into florets, and the frozen peas.
Add salt and pepper to taste. Serve the meat and the
vegetable soup separately.

Cotriade

3 onions
½ head fennel
3 tbsp polyunsaturated
  oil
1¾ pints (1 l) fish
  stock or water
½ tsp marjoram
½ tsp thyme
½ tsp chervil
1 bay leaf
2 tsp salt
pepper
½ bunch parsley
8 large potatoes
2½ lb (1.1 kg) fish
  (different types)
red wine vinegar
crushed peppercorns

Chop the onions and fennel and fry them in the oil over a low heat until the onion is transparent. Place the onion and fennel in a large saucepan and pour over the fish stock or water. Add the herbs, salt and pepper and the coarsely chopped parsley. Bring to the boil and add the peeled and sliced potatoes. Allow to simmer on a low fire for 10-12 minutes.

Clean the fish, chop them into pieces and add to the pan. Simmer for a further 10-12 minutes. Serve each person with a bowl of vinegar and crushed peppercorns in which to dip the fish pieces, and a small plate for the bones.

Potato and Leek Soup

5-6 medium-sized
  potatoes
3-4 leeks
1¾ pints (1 l) water or
  beef stock
5-8 peppercorns
salt

Peel and dice the potatoes, rinse the leeks and slice them into rings. Pour the stock or water into a pan, add the potatoes, leeks and peppercorns. Boil for about an hour or until the potatoes can be easily mashed. If a smoother consistency is desired, the soup can be whipped with an electric mixer. Add salt to taste.

This is a thick, filling soup and should be served piping hot with home-made wholewheat bread.

A good variation is to add a cauliflower, broken into florets, after 30 minutes' boiling time has passed, together with an onion cut in thin slices.

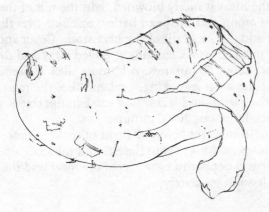

Salads

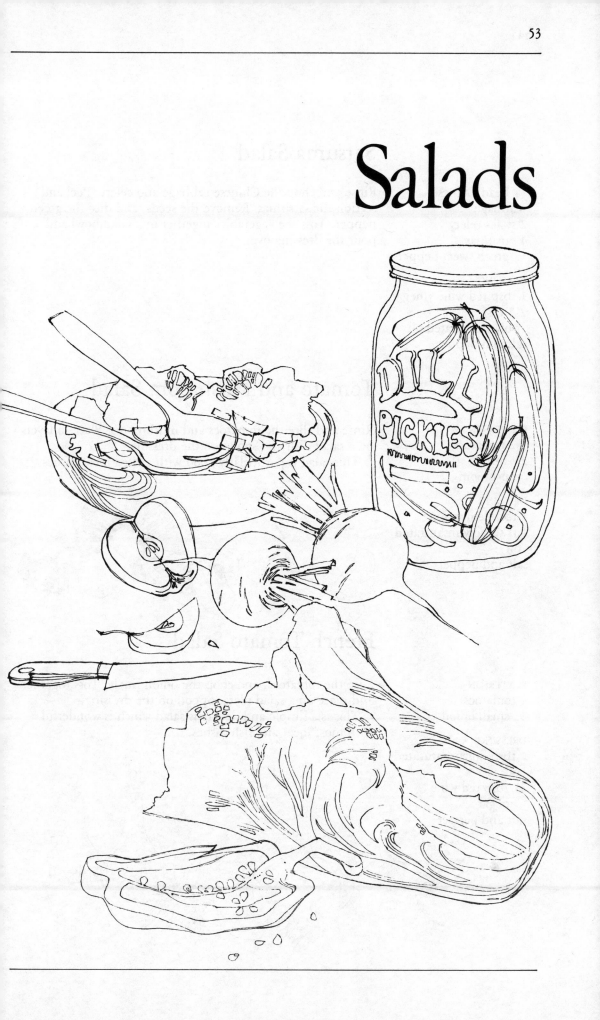

Satsuma Salad

½ head Chinese
  cabbage
2 stalks celery
4 satsumas
½ green sweet pepper

DRESSING
1 tbsp red wine vinegar
2-3 tbsp
  polyunsaturated oil
salt and pepper

Rinse and chop the Chinese cabbage and celery. Peel and section the satsumas. Remove the seeds, and dice the green pepper. Toss the vegetables together in a salad bowl and pour the dressing over.

Tomato and Mushroom Salad

PER PERSON
1-2 tomatoes
2½ oz (71 g)
  mushrooms

DRESSING
1 tbsp lemon juice
1 tbsp polyunsaturated
  oil
salt and pepper

Rinse and slice the tomatoes and mushrooms. Place in layers on a salad dish and spoon on the dressing.
  This salad is particularly good with grilled meat dishes.

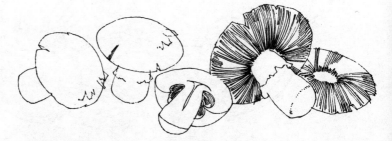

French Tomato Salad

PER PERSON
2 tomatoes
½ small onion

DRESSING
1 tbsp polyunsaturated
  oil
½ tbsp red wine
  vinegar
salt and pepper

Slice the tomatoes, and chop the onion finely, Toss together and place on a salad plate. Spoon on the dressing.
  This is a simple and delicious salad which is wonderful with most meat and fish dishes.

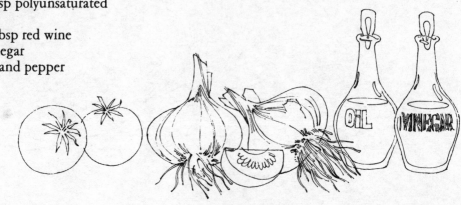

Bean Sprout Salad

1 lettuce
1 red sweet pepper
3 stalks celery
radishes
1 carrot
4 tomatoes
bean sprouts

DRESSING
juice of 1 lemon
3 tbsp polyunsaturated
   oil
2 cloves garlic (pressed)
1 tsp oregano
chopped parsley
salt

Shred the lettuce and cut the pepper into long strips. Slice the celery, radishes and carrot, and cut the tomatoes into wedges. Toss together with the bean sprouts in a large bowl. Mix the dressing and pour over the salad. Allow the salad to stand in a cool place for a while before serving.

Bean sprouts are easily grown in the home by following these instructions:

Take 2 tbsp of mung beans, rinse well in a strainer and place them in a glass jar. Fasten a piece of nylon net over the mouth of the jar with a rubber band. Fill the jar with water, and let the beans soak overnight. Drain, add fresh water to rinse them and pour it out again. (Leave the net on all the time.) Rinse the beans in this manner twice a day. They should be kept damp but not wet. In just a few days the bean sprouts are ready to eat.

Sprouts may be grown in this fashion from lentils, soy beans, wheat kernels, alfalfa seeds, etc.

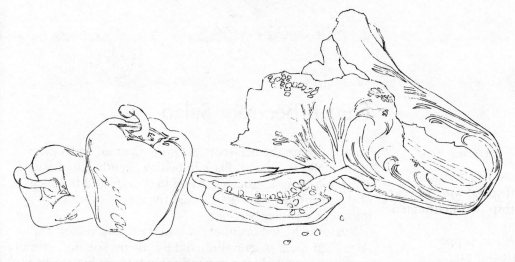

Avocado and Grapefruit Salad

2 PERSONS
1 avocado
1 grapefruit

DRESSING
1 tbsp polyunsaturated
   oil
½ tbsp red wine
   vinegar
salt

Cut the avocado into wedge-shaped slices and remove the skin. Peel the grapefruit and divide it into sections. Distribute the two fruits equally on two small dishes and pour on the dressing.

This salad is very good as a first course.

Mexican Orange and Cucumber Salad

1 cucumber
2 oranges
1 lettuce heart

MARINADE
5 tbsp polyunsaturated
  oil
3 ½ tbsp red wine
  vinegar
salt

DRESSING
2 tbsp marinade
2 tbsp orange juice
1 tbsp chili powder
salt

Slice the cucumber and place it in a bowl. Pour over the marinade, and leave to stand in a cool place for at least an hour.

Peel and slice the oranges, and shred the lettuce. Remove the cucumber from the marinade (save 2 tbsp of the marinade for the dressing). Toss the oranges, cucumber and lettuce in a bowl and pour over the dressing.

This salad is very good with meat or chicken dishes.

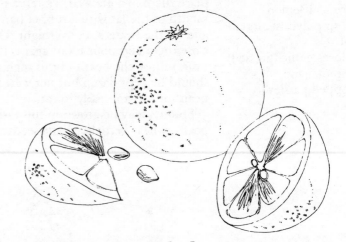

French Beetroot Salad

4-8 beetroots

VINAIGRETTE SAUCE
2 tbsp red wine vinegar
4 tbsp polyunsaturated
  oil
salt and pepper
¼ tsp sugar

Trim and rinse the beetroots, allowing the root and a piece of the stalks to remain. Place in boiling, lightly salted water. The cooking time varies according to the size and freshness of the beetroot. Allow 30 minutes for summer and 45 minutes for winter beetroots.

Rinse the boiled beetroots in cold water and rub off the skins. Cut them in thin slices and put them, still hot, in the vinaigrette sauce. Leave to stand for at least an hour. Serve them, perhaps with a spoonful of low fat cottage cheese, as an accompaniment to meat and fish dishes.

Balkan Cucumber Salad

1 cucumber
about 1 tsp salt
6 oz (170 g) low fat
  yogurt
ground black pepper

Peel the cucumber, cut into ¼-inch slices and quarter the slices. Place the pieces in a bowl and sprinkle on the salt. Allow to stand for 20 minutes, then pour off the liquid that has formed in the bottom of the bowl. Stir in the yogurt and black pepper and chill for a few hours before serving.

This recipe may be varied by pressing 1 clove of garlic into the yogurt or by adding thinly sliced onion.

Swedish Winter Salad

8 oz (226 g) red
cabbage
3 ½ oz (100 g)
cauliflower
1 apple
2 stalks celery
1 small leek
3 tbsp raisins

DRESSING
1 ½ tbsp
polyunsaturated oil
1 tbsp red wine vinegar
2 tbsp low fat yogurt
salt
½ tsp French mustard
(Dijon)

Shred the cabbage and break the cauliflower into florets.
Chop the apple and slice the celery and leek. Add the
raisins. Place everything in a large bowl, pour on the
dressing and toss.

This is a good and nutritious salad which goes well with
most meat and fish dishes.

Potato Salad

8-10 potatoes
1 leek
2-3 pickled beetroots
parsley
1 tbsp capers

SAUCE 1
2 tbsp polyunsaturated
oil
1 tbsp red wine vinegar
1 pinch tarragon
1 pinch garlic powder
salt and pepper

SAUCE 2
½ portion of sauce 1
2 tbsp low fat yogurt
½ tsp mustard or
tomato purée

Boil the potatoes in their skins. Meanwhile, mix the
ingredients for sauce 1. Peel the potatoes while they are still
hot, slice them, place in a bowl and pour over sauce 1.
Allow to cool. Before serving, carefully stir in the finely
sliced leek, diced beetroots, chopped parsley and capers. If
desired, chopped pickles and/or cocktail onions may be
added.

The salad may be served as it is or with a portion of sauce
2 poured over just before serving.

This salad is, without a doubt, best when fresh boiled
potatoes are used. If using left-over potatoes, either follow
the basic recipe or use only a double portion of sauce 2.

Parsnip Salad

2 large parsnips
5 oz (141 g) bean
  sprouts
5 tbsp chopped parsley

DRESSING
1½ tbsp
  polyunsaturated oil
1 tbsp red wine vinegar
3 tbsp low fat yogurt
salt and pepper

Peel the parsnips and coarsely grate them. Rinse the bean sprouts in a collander under cold running water, so that they become really crisp. Mix the ingredients together in a bowl and pour over the dressing.

Swedish Beetroot Salad

12 oz (340 g) boiled or
  pickled beetroots
1 large green apple
2 dill-pickled
  cucumbers
6-7 tbsp Mayonnaise
  (*see* p. 63)
salt and pepper

Dice the beetroots, the peeled and cored apples and the pickled cucumbers. Mix everything together in a bowl and add the mayonnaise, salt and pepper.

This salad is best as a light lunch served with rye bread and lean boiled ham, but can also be served as a side salad with meat or fish dishes.

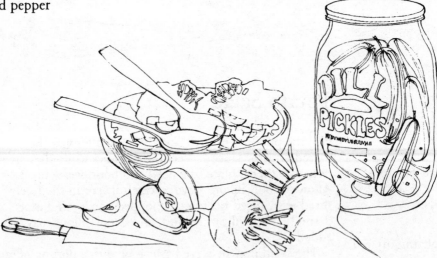

Sunny Salad

3 oranges
2 large carrots
3 tbsp raisins
2 tbsp chopped walnuts

Peel and dice the oranges. Peel and grate the carrots. Mix together in a bowl and add the raisins and walnuts.

This is a very simple but delicious salad.

Bean Salad

6 oz (170 g) red kidney
  beans
1 onion
1 green sweet pepper
1 7-oz (198-g) can
  sweet corn

DRESSING
2 tbsp polyunsaturated
  oil
1 tbsp red wine vinegar
salt and pepper

Soak the beans overnight; change the water and boil for
about an hour. Allow to cool.

Chop the onion, dice the green pepper and place them in
a large salad bowl. Add the cold beans and sweet corn, stir
and pour on the dressing.

This salad is very good with meat or chicken but can also
be served alone as a quick lunch together with home-made
bread.

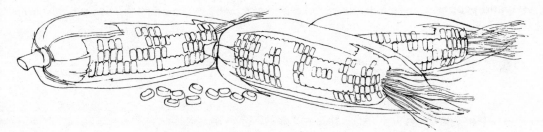

Salad Niçoise

4 boiled potatoes
1 onion
10 olives (black or
  green)
2 tomatoes
1 6½-oz (184-g) can
  tuna fish
10 anchovies
1 lettuce heart
1 bunch chives

DRESSING
2 tbsp polyunsaturated
  oil
1 tbsp red wine
  vinegar
salt and pepper

Peel and slice the potatoes, and place them in a bowl with
half the dressing. Peel and slice the onion as thinly as
possible, stone and halve the olives and cut the tomatoes
into wedges. Drain the tuna fish and anchovies thoroughly.
Rinse the lettuce leaves and cut them into smaller pieces.

Cover the bottom of a wide salad bowl with lettuce.
Arrange the rest of the ingredients over the lettuce. Sprinkle
with chopped chives, and pour on the remainder of the
dressing. Serve immediately with fresh home-made bread.

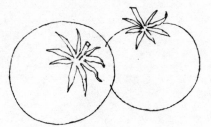

Chicory Salad

1 lb (454 g) walnuts
or
8 oz (226 g) shelled
  walnuts
8 heads chicory
1 grilled chicken

DRESSING
1 ½ tbsp red wine
  vinegar
3 tbsp polyunsaturated
  oil
salt and pepper

Mix the ingredients for the dressing and pour it over the shelled walnuts. Allow the nuts to steep in the dressing for a while. Rinse the chicory well and cut into strips lengthwise. Remove the skin and all visible fat from the grilled chicken and dice the meat. Toss the chicken meat and chicory in the dressing with the walnuts. This simple but delicious salad is perfect as a lunch or a light supper.

Sauces

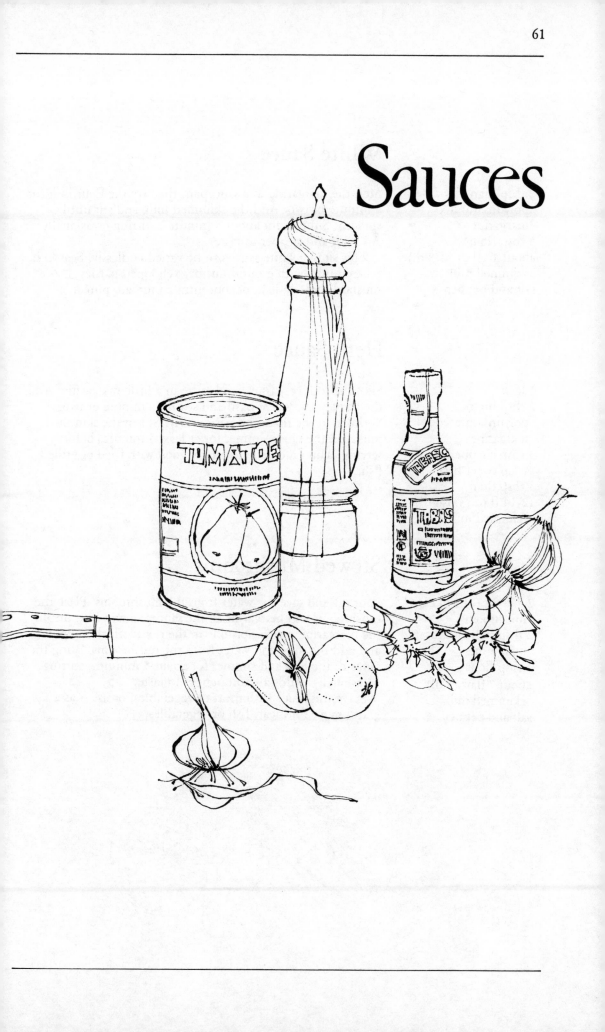

White Sauce

2 tbsp high-
  polyunsaturated
  margarine
5 tbsp flour
about 17 fl oz (4.8 dl)
  skimmed milk
salt and pepper

Melt the margarine in a saucepan, then fry the flour in it for
a minute or two. Add the skimmed milk and stir until
smooth. Simmer for about 5 minutes, stirring occasionally.
Add salt and pepper to taste.

    This simple white sauce can be varied endlessly. Season it,
for example, with ground nutmeg, chopped parsley,
mustard, horseradish, or concentrated tomato purée.

Herb Sauce

1 leek
2 tbsp high-
  polyunsaturated
  margarine
3 tbsp chopped parsley
¾ tsp sweet basil
3 tbsp flour
12-14 fl oz (3.5-4 dl)
  skimmed milk

Slice the leek very finely and sauté in a little margarine. Add
the parsley and sweet basil and stir for a minute or two.
Sprinkle in the flour and stir quickly. Stir in the skimmed
milk. Let the sauce simmer for at least 5 minutes before
serving. This sauce is particularly good with fried or grilled
fish.

Stewed Mushrooms

2 7½-oz (213-g) cans
  mushrooms
2 tbsp polyunsaturated
  margarine
4 tbsp flour
about 7 fl oz (2 dl)
  skimmed milk
salt and pepper

Pour off and save the water from the mushrooms. Place the
mushrooms and margarine in the saucepan and heat until
the margarine melts. Sprinkle in the flour, stir thoroughly,
and add the milk and water from the mushrooms. Bring the
sauce to the boil and simmer for about 5 minutes, stirring
occasionally. Add salt and pepper to taste.

    Serve this sauce with meat or vegetables; or use it as a
gratin sauce for meat, fish or vegetables.

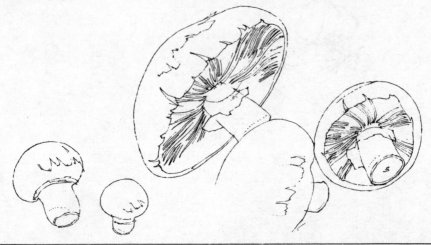

Mayonnaise

1 egg
3 tsp red wine vinegar
2 tsp mustard
14-18 fl oz (4-5 dl)
   polyunsaturated oil
salt and pepper

Beat the egg thoroughly in a bowl. Add the vinegar and mustard. Continue to whip the mixture rapidly while dripping the oil slowly into the bowl. Continue beating until the mayonnaise has the right thick, creamy texture. Salt and pepper to taste. This recipe yields abouts 18 fl oz of mayonnaise.

Cottage Cheese with Herbs

8 oz (226g) low fat
   cottage cheese
2 cloves garlic
chopped chives
chopped parsley
¼ tsp oregano
salt

Place the cottage cheese in a bowl, crush the garlic into it, add the chives, parsley and oregano, and stir. Salt to taste. Cottage cheese with herbs can be used instead of sauce with meat and fish dishes. It is also delicious as a sandwich spread or as a filling for baked potatoes.

Guacamole

1 avocado
5 fl oz (1.4 dl) low fat
   yogurt
2 tbsp lemon juce
pinch cayenne pepper

Cut the avocado in half, peel it and remove the stone. Mash the avocado in a bowl. Add the other ingredients and stir until thoroughly mixed. Serve the guacamole on a lettuce leaf, or use it as a dressing on a mixed salad, as a starter or a side salad.

Versatile Tomato Sauce

1 onion
2 cloves garlic
1 tbsp polyunsaturated
   oil
1 14-oz (397-g) can
   tomatoes
salt and pepper
2 tbsp wine or lemon
   juice, or 1 tbsp red
   wine vinegar
2 drops tabasco
¼ tsp sweet basil

Peel the onion and garlic, chop very finely, and sauté them in the oil for a minute or two. Pour on the tomatoes and bring to the boil. Mash the tomatoes with a fork and boil until the sauce has a thick smooth consistency. Add the salt, pepper and the wine or lemon juice or vinegar.

Choose spices according to how you intend to use the sauce. Tabasco and sweet basil, for example, make a good combination. But try other variants too, such as Worcestershire sauce, a good chili powder, bay leaves, thyme or curry powder.

After adding the seasoning of your choice, allow the sauce to simmer for a few minutes to bring out the true flavour of the spices.

This sauce is delicious with all kinds of pasta dishes and grilled meats. It is also excellent as a base for stews and soups.

Houmous

3 oz (85g) chick peas
3½ fl oz (1 dl) water (from boiling chick peas)
4 tbsp polyunsaturated oil
2 cloves garlic
salt

Soak the chick peas overnight. Drain, and add fresh cold water. Boil the peas in a covered pan for about 45 minutes, strain and cool. Grind the peas to a purée in a mincer or blender. Add the water from boiling the chick peas, the oil and crushed garlic. Salt to taste, and mix well. This recipe gives about 8 fl oz of houmous.

Place a spoonful of houmous on a lettuce leaf, garnish with a slice of cucumber and serve as a first course or use as a sandwich spread. It can also be used to round off a plate of grated vegetables.

Salsa de Chili Rojo
Red Chili Sauce

10-12 red chili peppers
2 onions
polyunsaturated oil
2 5-oz (140-g) cans concentrated tomato purée
1 pint 7 fl oz (7.7 dl) water
1-2 cloves garlic
1½ tsp salt
1 tsp oregano
¼ tsp ground caraway seeds
1 tsp chili powder

Clean the chili peppers, remove the seeds, and chop the peppers into thin semi-circles. Sauté the chopped onions in a little oil until they are transparent, but do not brown them. Place the onions in a large saucepan. Put the chilis in the frying pan with the rest of the oil and turn them a few times before adding to the saucepan. Add the water, tomato purée, pressed garlic, salt and spices. Bring to the boil and allow to simmer for about 20 minutes.

If a hotter sauce is desired, add a few—12 at the most— chili seeds to the sauce before simmering.

This sauce may be kept indefinitely if frozen and will keep for months in the refrigerator.

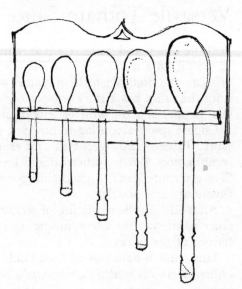

Vegetables

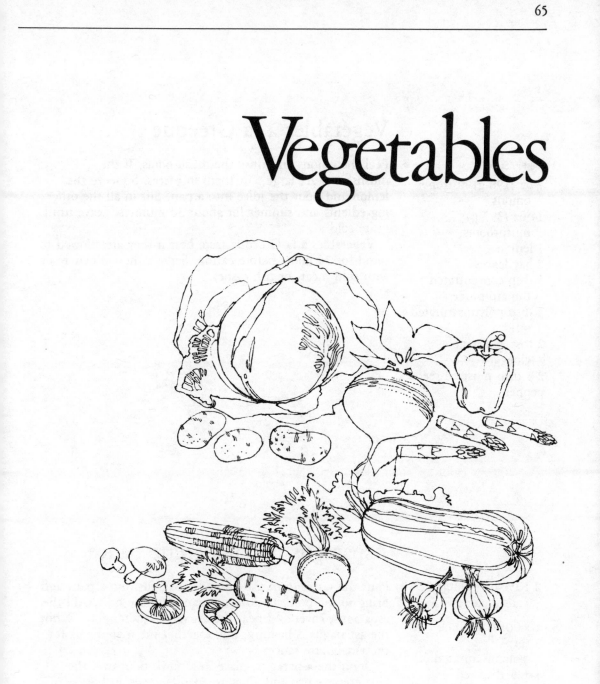

Vegetables à la Grecque

6-8 PERSONS

7 oz (198 g) button
  onions
14 oz (397 g)
  mushrooms
1 lemon
2 bay leaves
5 tbsp concentrated
  tomato purée
4 tbsp polyunsaturated
  oil
2 tbsp red wine
  vinegar
2-3 tbsp mustard seeds
pepper

Peel the onions and rinse the mushrooms. If the
mushrooms are large, cut them in pieces. Squeeze the
lemon and pour the juice into a pan. Stir in all the other
ingredients and simmer for about 30 minutes. Leave until
quite cold.

Vegetables à la Grecque taste best if they are allowed to
stand for 24 hours before eating. Serve as hors d'oeuvre or
with cold meat, or fish dishes.

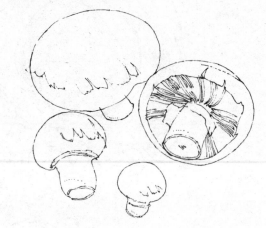

Asparagus in Vinaigrette Sauce

2 10½-oz (300 g)
  cans asparagus

VINAIGRETTE SAUCE
3 tbsp
  polyunsaturated oil
1-1½ tbsp red
  wine vinegar
¼ tsp chervil
1 tbsp chopped
  parsley
salt and pepper

Pour the water from the canned asparagus into a pan, and
bring to the boil. Remove the pan from the heat, add the
asparagus, cover and heat the asparagus thoroughly. While
the asparagus is heating, mix together the ingredients for
the vinaigrette sauce.

Drain the asparagus, place in a bowl, pour over the
vinaigrette sauce and allow to cool. Serve as an hors
d'oeuvre or as a complement to meat or fish.

This recipe may be varied by substituting haricots verts
or boiled leeks for asparagus.

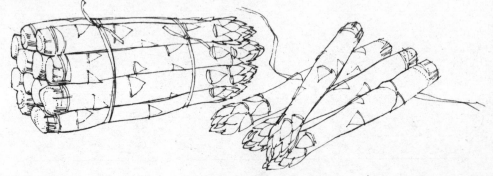

Braised Chicory

4-6 heads chicory
salt and pepper
about 5 fl oz (1.4 dl)
  beef stock
1 tbsp soy sauce
2 tbsp red wine

Clean, rinse and drain the heads of chicory. Place them in a greased casserole, and season with salt and pepper.

Mix the beef stock with the soy sauce and wine, and pour into the casserole until the chicory is half covered with the liquid. Cook in a moderately hot oven, 400°F or Gas No 5 (200°C), for about 30 minutes. Turn the chicory once during this time. Serve with meat dishes. Celery can also be prepared in this manner, but cook for about 20 minutes only.

Baked Celeriac with Stewed Mushrooms

1 celeriac about 1½ lb
  (6.5 hg)
1 portion Stewed
  Mushrooms (see
  p. 62)

Peel the celeriac and cut it into ½-inch-thick slices. Boil these in lightly salted water for about 10 minutes. Prepare the stewed mushrooms.

Place the celeriac slices in a greased casserole and cover with the stewed mushrooms. Bake in a very hot oven, 475°F or Gas No 8 (250°C), until the mushrooms are golden brown (about 20 minutes).

This dish is very good as a first course or as a vegetable with meat or fish. Try preparing other vegetables in this way, for example parsnips or cauliflower.

French Peas

1 tbsp high-
  polyunsaturated
  margarine
1 8-oz (226 g) packet
  frozen peas
6-10 button onions
1 lettuce heart
1 tsp sugar
1 tsp salt
about 7 fl oz (2 dl)
  water
parsley

Place ½ tbsp margarine in a pan and add all the other ingredients except the parsley. The water should *not* cover the peas. Boil for about 10-15 minutes, after which time there should be virtually no water left. Stir in the remaining ½ tbsp of margarine and the chopped parsley.

Button onions can be replaced by ordinary onions if these are chopped finely and sautéd until transparent before adding the other ingredients.

Tagliatelle and Mushrooms

PER PERSON
tagliatelle
4 oz (113 g)
   mushrooms
polyunsaturated oil
salt and pepper
2 cloves garlic
few drops lemon juice

Use less tagliatelle than shown on the package, since this dish is best as a first course.

Boil the pasta as usual. Rinse and slice the mushrooms and brown them slowly in the polyunsaturated oil. Add salt and pepper and the pressed garlic when the mushrooms are golden brown. Squeeze a few drops of fresh lemon juice over, pour the mushrooms over the boiled tagliatelle and serve.

Stuffed Peppers

4 green sweet peppers
1 large aubergine
1 large onion
9 oz (225 g)
   mushrooms
polyunsaturated oil
salt and pepper
2 tbsp chopped parsley
½ tsp sweet basil
7 tbsp breadcrumbs
4 tbsp white wine

Try to get peppers that will stand on end. Cut a hole in the top of each pepper and remove the seeds. Chop the aubergine, onion and mushrooms finely and brown them in a little oil. Add salt and pepper. Remove from the heat and add the parsley, sweet basil and breadcrumbs. Stir until evenly mixed.

Stuff the peppers with this mixture, place in a greased casserole and pour 1 tbsp of white wine in each. Bake in a hot oven, 430°F or Gas No 6-7 (225°C) for 25-30 minutes.

Other ingredients may be used as a stuffing, for example tomatoes, sweet corn or brown rice; stewed mushrooms are also very good. Also, try stuffing tomatoes, onions or aubergines.

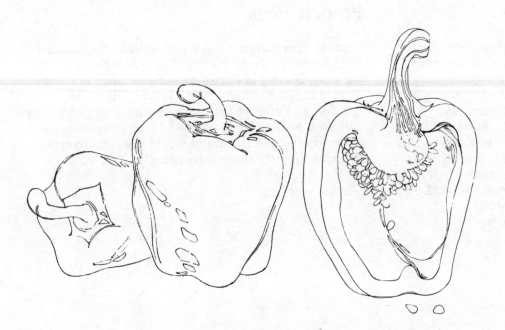

Fagotti

CRÈPES

3 oz (85 g) plain white
flour
½ tsp salt
10½ fl oz (3dl)
skimmed milk
3 tbsp dry white wine
(optional)
1 egg
1 egg white
2 tbsp high-
polyunsaturated
margarine

FILLING

1 6-oz (170 g) packet
frozen spinach
1 8-oz (226 g) carton
low fat cottage
cheese
¼ tsp ground nutmeg
salt
1 14-oz (397 g) can
tomatoes
¼ tsp garlic powder
1½ portions White
Sauce (see p. 62)
2 oz (56 g) vegetarian
cheese (optional)

Put the flour in a bowl and mix in the salt. Pour on a little of the liquid and beat to a smooth batter. Add the rest of the ingredients and continue beating. The margarine should be melted and allowed to cool before adding it to the batter. Fry about 8-10 thin crèpes.

Thaw the spinach and drain it well. Squeeze it in your hands to get all the water out. Mix the cottage cheese with the spinach and season with a little nutmeg and salt. Divide the mixture between the 8-10 crèpes and fold them into small packets or rolls.

Grease a casserole and spread half the tomatoes over the bottom. Dust with a little garlic powder and pour over half of the white sauce. Arrange the crèpes on top and cover them with slices of the vegetarian cheese, if this is to be used. Add the rest of the tomatoes, dust with more garlic powder, and cover with the remaining white sauce. Bake in a hot oven, 430°F, or Gas No 6-7 (225°C) for 10-12 minutes.

Ratatouille

4-6 PERSONS

3 aubergines
1 large onion
3 red sweet peppers
polyunsaturated oil
1 14-oz (397-g) can
tomatoes
½ tsp oregano
5-7 cloves garlic
salt and pepper
chopped parsley

Chop the aubergines, peeled onion and peppers. Sauté in a little oil in a heavy saucepan. Add the tomatoes, oregano and crushed garlic. Salt and pepper to taste. Cover and simmer for about 30 minutes, stirring occasionally. Sprinkle over plenty of chopped parsley before serving.

If ratatouille is served as a vegetable with meat or fish, this recipe is sufficient for 6 persons. However, it is also very good as a main dish served with Potato Casserole (see p. 75) brown rice or beans, and a salad, in which case the recipe is enough for 4 persons.

Spicy Baked Aubergine

2 PERSONS
1 aubergine about 8 oz
   (226 g)
4 oz (113 g)
   mushrooms
3 tbsp concentrated
   tomato purée
4 tbsp water
1 clove garlic
¼ tsp sweet basil
¼ tsp thyme
4 oz (113 g) low fat
   cottage cheese
2 tbsp breadcrumbs
1 tbsp high-
   polyunsaturated
   margarine

Boil the aubergine in lightly salted water for 10 minutes, making sure that it is completely submerged. Allow to cool and then cut it into ½-inch slices. Place the slices in a greased baking dish. Clean and slice the mushrooms and place them in a layer over the aubergine. Stir the tomato purée into the water, together with the pressed garlic and herbs. Pour the mixture over the mushrooms. Mix the cottage cheese with the breadcrumbs and spread over the top. Cook in a moderately hot oven, 400°F or Gas No 5 (200°C), for 25-30 minutes.

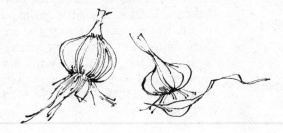

Onion Pie

PIE CRUST
6 oz (170 g) flour
pinch salt
3½ fl oz (1 dl)
   polyunsaturated oil
3 tbsp ice water

FILLING
3¼ lb (1.5 kg) onions
high-polyunsaturated
   margarine
salt and pepper

Mix the flour and salt in a bowl. Stir the oil and water together and pour over the flour. Mix to a dough and knead until it is smooth and shiny. Take about three quarters of the dough and roll out to a circle sufficient to cover the bottom and sides of a greased baking dish. Roll out the remaining dough thinly and cut into strips. Peel and slice the onions as thinly as possible. Fry slowly in a little margarine until soft and golden brown. Add salt and pepper. Place the onions in the pie shell and lay the dough strips over to form a lattice. Bake in a moderately hot oven, 400°F or Gas No 5 (200°C), for about 50 minutes or until the pie has a deep golden brown colour.

Potato Pancakes

10-12 potatoes
1 onion
1 tbsp skimmed milk
1 tsp salt
pepper
high-polyunsaturated
 margarine

Peel and coarsely grate the potatoes and onion. Mix together with the milk and seasoning. Heat a little margarine in a frying pan over a medium heat. Drop spoonfuls of the batter into the pan and spread them out into pancakes. Fry the potato pancakes, turning them once, until a beautiful brown on both sides.

Vegetarian Cabbage Rolls

1 cabbage about
 2 lb (9 hg)
1¾ pints (1 l) water
2 tsp salt

FILLING
1 onion
8 oz (226 g)
 mushrooms
2 tbsp polyunsaturated
 oil
salt and pepper
4 oz (113 g) boiled
 chopped cabbage
1 lb (454 g) boiled rice

SAUCE
10½-14 fl oz (3-4 dl)
 tomato juice
1 tsp salt
¼ tsp sweet basil or
 oregano
¼ tsp black pepper

Cut away as much as possible of the cabbage stalk. Place the cabbage head in the boiling salted water and boil for 10 minutes. Remove and allow to cool. Remove the larger leaves by cutting the base of each leaf and peeling it off. The small inner leaves are used in the filling and should be chopped. Chop the onion and mushrooms and fry them in the oil. Salt and pepper to taste. Stir in the chopped cabbage and the boiled rice. Place about 2 tbsp of the filling on each cabbage leaf and fold or roll into a little packet. Place the packets close together in a greased baking dish with the flap downwards. Mix the tomato juice with the salt, herbs and pepper and pour over the cabbage rolls. Cover the dish with aluminium foil and bake in a moderately hot oven, 400°F or Gas No 5 (200°C), for about an hour.

This recipe may be varied by using barley pilaff as a filling. It should then be mixed with raw chopped mushrooms.

Chick Pea Rissoles

ABOUT 16 RISSOLES
12 oz (340 g) chick
 peas
3 oz (85 g) brown rice
1 onion
salt and pepper
wholewheat flour
paprika powder to
 taste
polyunsaturated oil

Soak the chick peas overnight. Drain, and boil in fresh water for about 45 minutes. Boil the brown rice with 9 fl oz (2.5 dl) water in a small pan for about 40 minutes. Chop the onion very finely. Grind the chick peas in a mincer or purée them in a blender, and stir together with the brown rice and onion. Salt and pepper the mixture. Shape into patties and toss them in wholewheat flour mixed with paprika powder. Fry until golden brown in a little oil.

Serve with a salad or a selection of grated raw vegetables, for example carrots, beetroot, swedes, cabbage etc. The patties may be frozen raw and fried without thawing.

Carrot Rissoles

ABOUT 16 RISSOLES
5 oz (142 g) soy beans
1 lb (454 g) carrots
1 onion
5 tbsp water (from
   boiling the beans)
salt
wholewheat flour
high-polyunsaturated
   margarine

Soak the beans overnight. Drain, and boil in fresh water for about 45 minutes.

Grind the beans in a mincer or purée them in a blender. Mince the carrots very finely. Peel and chop the onion. Mix the bean mash, carrots and onion in a large bowl. Add enough water (from boiling the beans) to the mixture so that patties can be formed. Be careful not to use too much water. Salt to taste.

Shape into patties and toss them in the wholewheat flour. Fry in a little margarine until they are a golden brown.

The rissoles are delicious hot, but are also very good cold and are perfect for lunch boxes.

Celeriac Rissoles

ABOUT 16 RISSOLES
1 large celeriac about
   1½ lb (6.5 hg)
4 potatoes
salt
1 onion
breadcrumbs
polyunsaturated oil

Peel and slice the celeriac. Peel and dice the potatoes. Boil the celeriac and potatoes in lightly salted water. Mince the onion. Press the potatoes and celeriac through a vegetable mill or mash with a fork. Fold the onion into the mash. If the mixture is too dry add a little of the water used in boiling, but be careful not to let it become too mushy. Taste, and add more salt if needed. Shape into patties, toss them in the breadcrumbs, and fry in oil until golden brown.

Parsley Potatoes en Casserole

8-10 large potatoes
4 tbsp chopped parsley
salt and pepper
12 fl oz (3.5 dl) beef
   stock
2 tbsp high-
   polyunsaturated
   margarine

Peel the potatoes, cut into thick slices and place in a greased baking dish. Sprinkle parsley, salt and pepper between the layers and on top.

Boil the beef stock and add the margarine. Pour the mixture carefully into the dish so as not to wash away the parsley. Cover with aluminium foil and bake in a hot oven, 430°F or Gas No 6-7 (225°C), for about 45 minutes.

Better Beans

6-8 PERSONS

12 oz (340 g) haricot
  beans
1-2 onions
5-7 cloves
2-3 bay leaves
1 tbsp polyunsaturated
  oil
1 clove garlic
  (optional)
2 pints 13 fl oz (1.5 l)
  water
1-2 tsp salt

TOMATO SAUCE
1 small onion
1 clove garlic
1 tbsp polyunsaturated
  oil
12 fl oz (3.4 dl)
  tomato juice
4 tbsp concentrated
  tomato purée
1 tsp salt
pepper
¼ tsp thyme
3-4 drops
  Worcestershire sauce
1 drop tabasco
parsley

Soak the beans for at least 6 hours — preferably overnight.
Pour off the water and place the beans in a large saucepan.
Add the onions, peeled and stuck with the cloves, the bay
leaves, oil and garlic. Add the water and boil on a low heat
for 1-1½ hours. Add the salt at the end of the cooking
time. Pour off the water and remove the bay leaves and
onions.

The beans are now ready and can be used as they are
with fish or meat, or in soups and salads. We suggest a
rich tomato sauce: mince the onion and fry with the
pressed garlic until transparent. Add the tomato juice and
purée, stir in the remaining ingredients, and simmer for a
few minutes before tasting. The sauce should be strong,
rich and racy. Add more spices if necessary. Stir in the
beans, heat gently until thoroughly hot and garnish with
chopped parsley.

Serve with green salad and home-made bread or as a
vegetable with grilled pork or lamb chops.

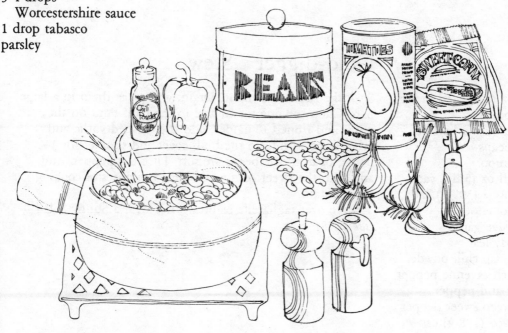

Vegetable Casserole

4-6 PERSONS
8 potatoes
8 Jerusalem artichokes
3 carrots
10 small onions
1 small swede
½ celeriac
1 parsnip
2 leeks

SAUCE
3½ fl oz (1 dl) tomato
  juice
2 tbsp concentrated
  tomato purée
2 tbsp soy sauce
1 tbsp red wine
  vinegar
½ tsp mustard powder
1 tsp salt
¼ tsp black pepper
1 crumbled bay leaf

Peel the vegetables and chop them into pieces. (The smaller the pieces, the shorter the cooking time.) Place the chopped vegetables in a greased baking dish. Stir together all the ingredients for the sauce and pour over the vegetables. Put the dish in a moderately hot oven, 400°F or Gas No 5 (200°C), for about an hour or until the vegetables are soft. Serve with brown rice and soy sauce or with barley pilaff (see p.75).

Try using other vegetables; choose according to taste and season. The variations are endless and they are all equally good.

Gold-digger's Stew

3 oz (85 g) red kidney
  beans
3 oz (85 g) haricot
  beans
1 onion
18 fl oz (5 dl) water
1 14-oz (397-g) can
  tomatoes
1 clove garlic
1 bay leaf
1½ tsp chili powder
pinch cayenne pepper
salt and pepper
1 green sweet pepper
1 7-oz (198-g) can
  sweet corn

Soak the beans overnight. Drain, and place them in a large pan. Chop the onion and add to the pan. Pour on the water and tinned tomatoes, add the crushed garlic and other spices. bring to the boil, cover and simmer for 1¼ hours, or until the beans are soft. Dice the pepper, and add with the sweet corn when only 5 minutes of cooking time remain.

Serve over tagliatelle or brown rice with a Sunny Salad (see p.58).

Pam's Nice Rice

1 onion
1 small sweet green
  pepper
polyunsaturated oil
1 14-oz (397-g) can
  tomatoes
6 oz (170 g) brown
  rice
7 fl oz (2 dl) water
salt

Chop the onion and green pepper very finely. Fry them lightly in a little oil in a large pan. Add the tomatoes, brown rice, water and salt. Cover and allow to cook slowly for about 45 minutes, stirring occasionally and adding water if necessary.

Potato Casserole

about 2 lb (9 hg)
  potatoes
1 large onion
salt and pepper
ground nutmeg
3-4 tbsp skimmed milk
1 tbsp high-
  polyunsaturated
  margarine

Peel and slice the potatoes. (If the skins are not too thick, it is sufficient to merely scrub them.) Peel and slice the onion. Place the potatoes, onion and spices in layers in a greased baking dish. Pour on the milk and add the margarine in small dabs over the surface. Bake in a hot oven, 430°F or Gas No 6-7 (225°C), for about an hour or until nicely browned.

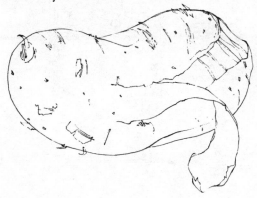

Barley Pilaff

4-6 PERSONS
6 oz (170 g) pearl
  barley
2 onions
¼ celeriac
1 carrot
3 tbsp polyunsaturated
  oil
1 tsp salt
¼ tsp thyme
1 pint 4 fl oz (7 dl)
  beef stock or water

Place the barley in a strainer and rinse well. Peel and chop the onions. Peel the celeriac and carrot and cut them into thin strips. Sauté the onions and vegetables in the oil until the onions are transparent. Put the onions and vegetables in a pan, add the barley, salt and thyme. Pour over the beef stock or water. Cover and boil on a low heat for about 45 minutes.
    Serve with meat or fish or with stewed mushrooms.

Exotic Lentil Curry

1-2 onions
1 small carrot
polyunsaturated oil
3-4 tsp curry powder
1 pint 3 fl oz (6-7 dl)
  water
6 oz (170 g) red lentils
3 tbsp soy sauce
1 potato
1 lb (454 g)
  mushrooms
1 small leek
1 banana
2 apples
½ tsp ginger

Peel and chop the onions, slice the carrot. Fry the onion and carrot together lightly in a little oil. Sprinkle the curry powder over the vegetables in the frying pan and stir together for a minute or two. Place in a saucepan, add the water, lentils and soy sauce. Peel and dice the potato and add to the pan. Boil for about 35 minutes, stirring occasionally.

While the lentils are cooking, slice the mushrooms, leek and banana, and dice the apple. Sprinkle the apple with ginger and fry everything lightly in a little oil. Add to the pan for the last ten minutes of cooking time.

Serve with brown rice, bread and a salad.

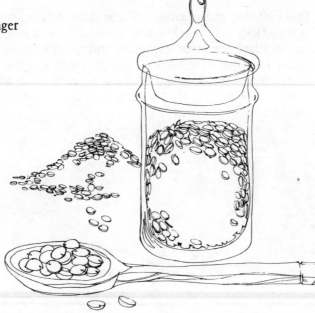

Fish

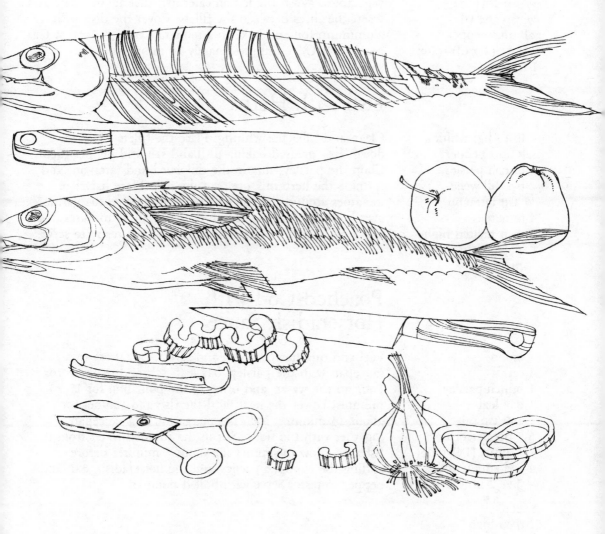

Lemon Whiting

2 ½ lb (1.1 kg) whiting
1 onion
1 carrot
1 leek
1 stalk celery
1 small bunch parsley
1 bay leaf
¼ tsp thyme
½ tsp chervil
salt and pepper
9 fl oz (2.5 dl) water
1 lemon

Clean, rinse and fillet the whiting. Peel, rinse and chop the vegetables, place them together with the herbs in a saucepan and pour on the water. Cover, and boil slowly for about 15 minutes. Remove the lid and allow the stock to boil down to concentrate the flavour.

Season the whiting fillets with salt and pepper and put them in a greased baking dish. Pour over the stock and vegetables. Wash the lemon carefully, slice it cross-wise and insert the slices between the fillets. Cover the dish with aluminium foil and bake in a moderate oven, 375°F or Gas No 4 (200°C), for approximately 20 minutes.

Fish with Herbs

2 lb (9 hg) whiting
salt and pepper
1 bunch parsley
2 tsp dill weed
½ tsp tarragon
4 tomatoes
3 tbsp melted high-polyunsaturated margarine

Clean and fillet the whiting. Place the fillets, skin side down, in a greased baking dish and salt and pepper them. Chop the parsley, mix in the dill weed and tarragon, and sprinkle the herb mixture over the fish. Place halves of tomatoes around the fish and pour the melted margarine over both the fish and tomatoes. After 30-35 minutes in a hot oven, 425°F or Gas No 6 (225°C), it is ready to serve.

Poached Cod with Horseradish Sauce

1 onion
1 carrot
1 bunch parsley
1 bay leaf
1-1½ tsp salt
6-7 peppercorns
1¾ pints (1 l) water
4 cod cutlets about
    1½-2 lb (6.5-9 hg)

SAUCE
2 tbsp high-polyunsaturated margarine
5 tbsp flour
14-18 fl oz (4-5 dl) fish stock
chopped parsley
2 tsp grated horseradish

Peel and quarter the onion and carrot, put them in a saucepan with the parsley, bay leaf, salt and peppercorns. Pour on the water, and bring to the boil. Boil for 15-20 minutes. Lower the heat, add the fish and simmer for about 15 minutes. Melt the margarine in a saucepan together with the flour. Stir in the strained water from the fish and allow to simmer for about 5 minutes before adding the chopped parsley and the horseradish. Salt and pepper to taste. Serve with boiled potatoes.

Cod Florentine

PER PERSON
8 oz (226 g) spinach
½ small onion
1-2 tomatoes
6-8 oz (170-226 g) cod
   fillet
salt and pepper
breadcrumbs
high-polyunsaturated
   margarine

Cook the spinach in lightly salted boiling water for about 5 minutes. Chop the onion and tomatoes.

Salt and pepper the cod fillet and toss it in the breadcrumbs. Fry in a little margarine and place on a bed of drained spinach. Garnish with the onion and tomatoes.

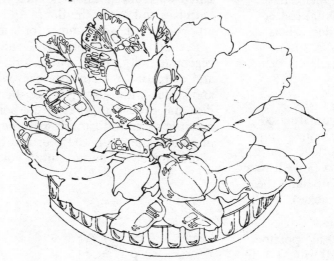

Turbot Papilotte

4-5 PERSONS
1 large turbot about
   2-2½ lb
   (9 hg-1.1 kg)
2 tbsp high-
   polyunsaturated
   margarine
salt and pepper
8 oz (226 g)
   mushrooms
8 oz (226 g) spring
   onions
1 bunch parsley
7 fl oz (2 dl) dry white
   wine

Clean the fish and cut into 4-5-inch-thick slices. Melt one tbsp of the margarine in a frying pan and fry the slices for a few minutes on each side, sprinkling them with salt and pepper. Put the fried fish to one side.

Rinse the mushrooms, peel the onions and chop them with parsley as finely as possible. Fry the mixture for a minute or two in a frying pan, using the rest of the margarine. Season with salt and pepper and pour on the wine. Bring to the boil and simmer for a few minutes. Divide the fried mushrooms and onions evenly between 4-5 sheets of baking parchment or oiled greaseproof paper and place a slice of fish on each mound of mushrooms. Fold the paper carefully into a tight packet, paying particular attention to the edges to ensure the packet is as airtight as possible. Place the packets on a baking sheet and bake in a moderately hot oven, 400°F or Gas No 5 (200°C), for 10-12 minutes.

Serve each person an unopened packet.

Baked Fish with Jerusalem Artichokes

1 onion
1 bay leaf
salt
6-7 peppercorns
2 lb (9 hg) cod or
  haddock fillets
1½ lb (6.8 hg)
  Jerusalem artichokes

SAUCE
2 tbsp high-
  polyunsaturated
  margarine
4 tbsp flour
14 fl oz (3.9 dl) water
  (from boiling the
  artichokes)

MASHED POTATOES
2 lb (9 hg) potatoes
3½-5 fl oz (1-1.5 dl)
  skimmed milk
1 tbsp high-
  polyunsaturated
  margarine
salt and pepper
ground nutmeg

Boil together the chopped onion, bay leaf, salt and peppercorns. Add the fish and allow to simmer for 5 minutes. Peel the Jerusalem artichokes and boil in lightly salted water for 20 minutes. Melt the margarine in a saucepan and stir in the flour. Add the water from the artichokes. Stir, and simmer for 5 minutes.

Peel and boil the potatoes. Drain and press in a vegetable mill or mash with a fork. Add the skimmed milk and margarine and stir together. Salt and pepper to taste and season with nutmeg. Place the fish in a greased baking dish and cover with slices of the boiled artichokes. Pour over the sauce and garnish with the mashed potatoes. Bake in a moderate oven, 400°F or Gas No 5 (200°C), for approximately 20 minutes until golden brown.

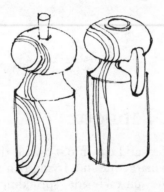

Pimento Plaice

2 PERSONS
1 small onion
1 14-oz (397-g)
  can pimentos
high-polyunsaturated
  margarine
2 tbsp concentrated
  tomato purée
3½ fl oz (1 dl) white
  wine
1 clove garlic
salt and pepper
12 oz (340 g) plaice
chopped parsley

Peel and chop the onion and dice the pimentos. Sauté the onions in a pan in a little margarine, and add the pimentos, tomato purée, wine and pressed garlic. Salt and pepper to taste and allow to simmer for about 15 minutes.

Salt and pepper the plaice fillets and place them in a greased baking dish. Pour over the sauce and bake in a hot oven, 430°F or Gas No 6-7 (225°C), for about 35 minutes. Sprinkle with chopped parsley and serve.

Boiled potatoes or home-made brown bread, and a salad complete the meal.

Curry Covered Fish

1 onion
1 small carrot
a few sprigs parsley
8 white peppercorns
14 fl oz (4 dl) water
1 tsp salt
1½ lb (6.8 hg) cod or
  haddock fillets

SAUCE
1 tbsp high-
  polyunsaturated
  margarine
2 tbsp flour
about ½ pint (2.8 dl)
  stock from the
  boiled fish
3½ fl oz (1 dl)
  skimmed milk
2-3 onions
1 tbsp polyunsaturated
  oil
½ tsp curry powder
2 tomatoes
salt
1 tbsp breadcrumbs

Peel the onion and carrot and cut them into quarters. Place the vegetables in the water together with the parsley and peppercorns, and boil for 10 minutes. Then add the fish to the boiling water and simmer for 6-8 minutes. For the sauce, melt the margarine in a saucepan and stir in the flour. Fry for a minute before adding the fish stock and skimmed milk. Allow to boil for a few minutes, stirring continually. Peel and slice the onions and fry them in the oil until transparent. Sprinkle in the curry powder and fry for a few more minutes. Grease a baking dish and arrange the boiled fish fillets in the base. Cover with the curried onions, and then add a layer of thin tomato slices. Pour over the sauce and sprinkle with the breadcrumbs. Bake for 5 minutes in a very hot oven, 500°F or Gas No 9 (260°C). This recipe can be varied by using saffron instead of curry.

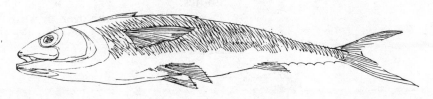

Salmon with Mushrooms and Herbs

2 lb (9 hg) salmon
1 onion
1 bunch parsley
1 bunch chives
1 bay leaf
1 tsp black
  peppercorns
¼ tsp thyme
1 tsp salt
3½ fl oz (1 dl)
  polyunsaturated oil
8 oz (226 g)
  mushrooms
high-polyunsaturated
  margarine

Cut the salmon in slices and place them in a greased baking dish. Chop the onion, parsley and chives, and crumble the bay leaf. Pound the peppercorns in a mortar, mix with spice and salt and sprinkle over the salmon. Pour on the oil and allow to stand in a cool place for about 3-6 hours.

Clean the mushrooms and fry them lightly in a little margarine. Drain off the oil from the salmon, top with the mushrooms and bake in a hot oven, 430°F or Gas No 6-7 (225°C), for about 20 minutes. The cooking time varies with the thickness of the salmon slices.

Serve with boiled potatoes and a salad. The salmon can be substituted by halibut if preferred.

Lemon Sole à la Monique

2 lemon sole (or plaice) about 2 ½ lb (1.1 kg)
1 onion
parsley
8 oz (226 g) mushrooms
salt and pepper
3 tbsp melted high-polyunsaturated margarine
breadcrumbs
7 fl oz (2 dl) dry white wine
2-4 tbsp madeira or sherry

Skin the fish on the darker upper side and scrape the skin on the lighter underside. Removing the skin can be difficult, so if you are not good at cleaning fish, ask your fishmonger to do this for you.

Chop the onion and parsley, and slice the mushrooms thinly. Make a bed of the onion, parsley and mushrooms in the bottom of a greased baking dish. Sprinkle with salt and pepper, and place the fish, skinned side up on the vegetables. Brush with the melted margarine and dust with salt, pepper and breadcrumbs. Pour the wines carefully into the dish but not over the fish (do not dislodge the breadcrumbs). The amount of liquid will vary with the size of dish, but should be sufficient to submerge the underside while the upper side with the breadcrumbs remains dry. If necessary, the wine may be diluted with water. Bake in a very hot oven, 500°F or Gas No 9 (260°C), until the fish are golden brown, about 10-15 minutes.

Serve direct from the oven or with White Sauce (*see* p. 62), made with liquid formed at the bottom of the onion and mushroom bed.

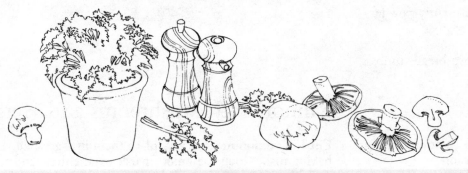

Granny's Fish Pudding

1 lb (454 g) cod or haddock fillets
7 fl oz (2 dl) water
½ tsp salt
3 oz (85 g) rice
9 fl oz (2.6 dl) skimmed milk
3 tbsp high-polyunsaturated margarine
1 egg yolk (optional)
salt and pepper
3 egg whites

Boil and mince the fish fillets. Bring the water to the boil, add the salt and rice, cover and simmer until the water has boiled off (about 20 minutes). Pour on the milk and simmer for a further 15 minutes, until you have a thin porridge. Stir in the margarine, fish and egg yolk (if used). Add salt and pepper if needed. Beat the egg whites until stiff, fold carefully into the porridge. Pour the batter into a greased casserole dish and bake in a very moderate oven, 350°F or Gas No 3, (175°C), for about 45 minutes.

Baccallao
Portuguese Sailor's Dish

8 potatoes
7 fl oz (2 dl) tomato
 juice
1 portion Versatile
 Tomato Sauce
 seasoned with sweet
 basil or thyme (*see*
 p. 63)
4-6 cod fillets
salt and pepper

Peel the potatoes and cut them into thin slices. Put the slices in a pan and boil them in the tomato juice for about 15 minutes. Check the liquid level from time to time.

Add the tomato sauce. Salt and pepper the cod fillets place them on top of the tomato sauce and simmer for a further 15 minutes.

Spanish Cod

3 lb (1.3 kg) cod fillets
salt and pepper
2 tbsb melted high-
 polyunsaturated
 margarine
1 clove garlic
parsley
¼ tsp tarragon
4 tbsp breadcrumbs

Slash shallow grooves about an inch apart diagonally across the skin side of the fillets. Salt and pepper the flesh side and place the fillets, flesh side down, in a greased baking dish. Brush the fish with the melted margarine. Mix the pressed garlic, chopped parsley and tarragon together and push it into the grooves in the skin side of the fillets. Sprinkle the breadcrumbs over the fish and bake in a very hot oven, 500°F or Gas No 9 (260°C) for about 10 minutes. Baste occasionally with the liquid that forms in the bottom of the dish.

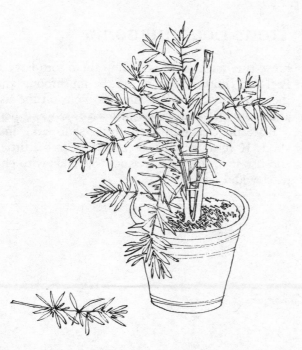

Baked Trout

PER PERSON
1 small trout
salt and pepper
1 tbsp chopped parsley
¼ tsp sweet basil
2 tbsp chopped onion
2 tbsp white wine

Clean the fish but leave the head and tail on. Salt and pepper the inside, and place the fish on a greased sheet of aluminium foil. Stuff the fish with a mixture of the parsley, sweet basil and onion, and spoon over the wine. Fold the foil together tightly and bake the fish in a moderately hot oven, 400°F or Gas No 5 (200°C), for 20 minutes. Serve with boiled potatoes and a fresh salad.

Marinated Trout

4 small trout
salt and pepper
wholewheat flour
high-polyunsaturated
    margarine

MARINADE
5 tbsp polyunsaturated
    oil
2 tbsp red wine
    vinegar
1 tbsp chopped parsley
1 small onion
1 clove garlic
salt and pepper

Clean and rinse the fish, and dry them carefully. Season with salt and pepper and toss in wholewheat flour. Fry in a little margarine, and leave until cold.

Make a marinade from the oil, vinegar, parsley, chopped onion, pressed garlic, salt and pepper. Place the fish in a suitable container and pour on the marinade. Let them steep for two days, turning once.

Remove the fish and drain on absorbent paper before serving. Serve with fresh home-made rye or barley bread and a good salad.

Trout Bourguignonne

2 PERSONS
4 oz (113 g)
    mushrooms
½ onion
1 tbsb high-
    polyunsaturated
    margarine
3½ fl oz (1 dl) fish
    stock
3½ fl oz (1 dl) red
    wine
a pinch of sage
salt and pepper
2 trout
1 tsp arrowroot
parsley

Rinse the mushrooms and chop them into large pieces. Peel and chop the onion. Fry the mushrooms and onion in the margarine for a few minutes. Pour on the fish stock and red wine, and season with sage, salt and pepper.

Place the cleaned trout into the sauce and simmer for about 10 minutes. Stir the arrowroot into a little cold water and use it to thicken the sauce. Sprinkle with chopped parsley and serve.

Grilled Mackerel

4 mackerel fillets
1 lemon
2 tbsp polyunsaturated
   oil
½ tsp fennel seeds
salt

Trim the fillets and skin them if this has not been done. Squeeze the lemon and mix the juice with the oil. Pour the oil and lemon juice mixture over the fillets, and let them steep for ½-1 hour.

Pound the fennel seeds in a mortar or grind finely. Remove the fish fillets from the oil and lemon mixture and dry them. Sprinkle with the powdered fennel seeds and salt, and grill for 3-4 minutes on each side.

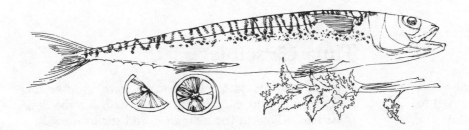

Caesar's Sole

2 lb (9 hg) fillet of
   sole
salt and pepper
1 small onion
chives
parsley
5 tomatoes
3½ fl oz (1 dl) dry
   white wine
1 tbsp white wine
   vinegar
1 clove garlic
1 tsp French mustard
   (Dijon)

SAUCE
 2 tbsp high-
   polyunsaturated
   margarine
1 tbsp flour
10½ fl oz (3 dl) fish
   stock
1 tsp concentrated
   tomato purée
1 tbsp breadcrumbs

Salt and pepper the fillets, fold in half and arrange in a greased baking dish. Chop the onion, chives and parsley. Peel the tomatoes and remove the seeds. Dice the tomato flesh. Set aside one tomato for garnishing.

Mix the wine and vinegar in a saucepan. Add 2 tbsp chopped parsley, 1 tbsp chopped chives, and the flesh from 4 tomatoes. Add the pressed garlic and stir in the mustard. Bring to the boil and pour over the fillets. Cover with aluminium foil and bake in a moderately hot oven, 400°F or Gas No 5 (200°C), for 20 minutes.

Melt the margarine in a saucepan together with the flour. Stir in the fish stock and simmer for a few minutes, stiring occasionally. Season with the tomato purée and salt and pepper if needed. Pour the sauce over the fish and sprinkle with breadcrumbs. Bake in a very hot oven, 500°F, or Gas No 9 (260°C) for 5 minutes. Garnish with diagonal stripes of chopped tomato flesh and chopped parsley. Serve with boiled potatoes.

Mackerel on Potato Cake

2 PERSONS
5 medium-sized
   potatoes
1 large onion
salt and pepper
high-polyunsaturated
   margarine
12 oz (340 g) cleaned
   smoked mackerel
chopped parsley

Peel the potatoes and grate them coarsely. Rinse under
running water and drain on absorbent paper. Peel the
onion and slice as thinly as possible. Mix with the grated
potatoes, season with salt and pepper and fry in a little
margarine over a low heat for about 30 minutes. Do not
stir.

Mince the mackerel, and when only 5 minutes of frying
time is left, sprinkle it over the potatoes together with the
chopped parsley.

Tuna Casserole

8 potatoes
about 2½ fl oz
   (0.7 dl)
   skimmed milk
1 tbsp high-
   polyunsaturated
   margarine
salt and pepper
nutmeg
2 6½-oz (285-g) cans
   tuna fish
½ onion
2-3 stalks celery
2 tbsp lemon juice
2 egg whites
2 tsp mustard or
   3 tbsp Mayonnaise
   (see p. 63)

Peel and boil the potatoes and mash them. Add boiling
milk, stirring continuously, until the mash has the desired
consistency. Fold in the margarine and stir in the salt,
pepper and a little nutmeg. Drain the tuna thoroughly and
mince it. Peel and chop the onions as finely as possible.
Chop the celery and stir the celery, tuna, onion and lemon
juice into the mashed potatoes. Place the mixture in a
greased baking dish.

Stiffly beat the egg whites and carefully fold in the
mustard or mayonnaise. Spread the egg mixture over the
mash and bake in a very moderate oven, 350°F or Gas
No 3 (175°C), for about 30 minutes.

Serve immediately with a crisp salad.

Mustard Crusted Sprats

2 lb (9 hg) sprats
1 egg
4 tbsp mustard
wholewheat flour
salt
high-polyunsaturated
   margarine

Clean the sprats (see illustration). Rinse the fillets and let
them drain thoroughly. Whip the egg in a bowl and beat
in the mustard. Put the sprats into the mixture and set
aside to stand in a cool place for a few hours.

Mix the wholewheat flour with salt and turn the fish in
this. Fry the sprats in a little margarine until golden
brown. Serve with boiled or mashed potatoes and a green
salad.

This is an inexpensive and delicious dish. Naturally,
Baltic Herring may be used if preferred.

Tomato Sprats

2 lb (9 hg) sprats
salt and pepper

TOMATO MARINADE
4 tbsp concentrated
   tomato purée
4 tbsp water
2 tbsp polyunsaturated
   oil
1 tbsp red wine
   vinegar
salt and pepper

Clean and rinse the sprats and allow to drain. Salt and pepper the inside of each fish, fold in half with the back up, and place side by side in a saucepan.

Mix the ingredients for the tomato marinade together and pour over the fish. Bring to the boil and simmer for about 7 minutes.

Serve the fish either hot or cold with boiled potatoes. If cold, the fish is also very good in sandwiches.

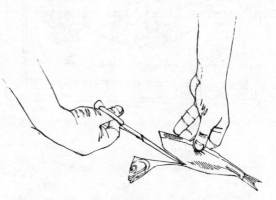

1. Using sharp scissors, cut behind the head without completely removing it.

2. Continue cutting right along the stomach.

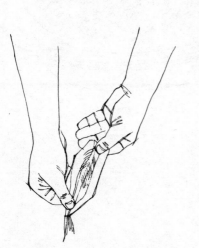

3. Pull your thumb along the back-bone unfolding the fish and removing the guts.

4. Pull out the bone.

Fowl

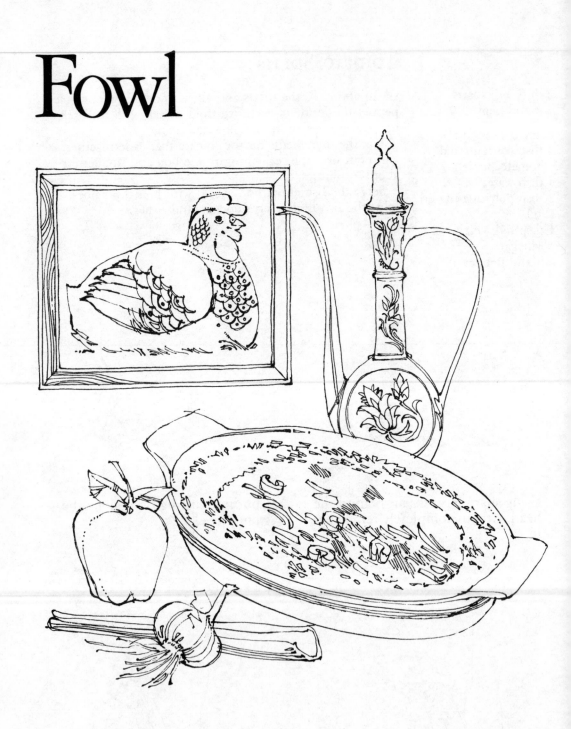

Chicken in the Pot

1 chicken about 3 lb
  (1.3 kg)
1½ tsp salt
¼ tsp tarragon
1 clove garlic
2 bunches parsley
1 onion
3 stalks celery

SAUCE
3 tbsp concentrated
  tomato purée
3 tbsp soy sauce
1 tbsp red wine
  vinegar
¼ tsp tarragon
2 cloves garlic

Dry the chicken well. Mix together the salt, tarragon and pressed garlic, and rub the chicken with the mixture both inside and out. Chop the parsley and stuff the chicken with it. Peel and slice the onion and chop the celery. Make a bed of the vegetables in the bottom of a chicken brick and place the chicken on this.

Mix the tomato purée, soy sauce, vinegar, tarragon and pressed garlic. Pour the sauce over the chicken, and cover. Put the brick into the cold oven, and set the oven at 500°F or Gas No 9 (260°C). Cooking time is about 1 hour and 45 minutes.

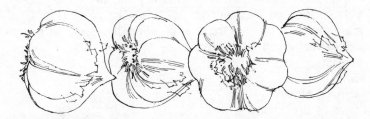

Chicken à la Diable

1 chicken about 2½ lb
  (1.1 kg)
salt and pepper
2 tbsp melted high-
  polyunsaturated
  margarine

SAUCE
4 peppercorns
5 fl oz (1.4 dl) chicken
  stock
6 fl oz (1.7 dl) white
  wine
1½ tbsp white wine
  vinegar
2 tbsp chopped
  onion
¼ tsp tarragon
1 tsp concentrated
  tomato purée
2-3 tsp French mustard
  (Dijon)
1½ tsp arrowroot

Dry the bird carefully and tie the legs together. Salt and pepper to taste, and brush with the melted margarine. Place the chicken on a grid, set over a roasting tin, in a very moderate oven, 350°F or Gas No 3 (175°C), for 1¼ hours. Cover with aluminium foil towards the end of the baking time if the chicken becomes too brown. Add no liquid at all. Crush the peppercorns and mix all the ingredients except the arrowroot in a saucepan. Simmer for 7-8 minutes. Thicken with the arrowroot dissolved in a little cold water. Strain the sauce to remove the peppercorns.

This dish is very good served with brown rice and a crisp green salad.

Chicken Montezuma

1½ tsp chili powder
½ tsp ground cloves
¼ tsp ground caraway
 seeds
½ tsp black pepper
1½ tsp salt
1 chicken about 2½ lb
 (1.1 kg)
2 oz (56 g) lean
 smoked ham
parsley
2 cloves garlic
1 tbsp melted high-
 polyunsaturated
 margarine
1 small sweet green
 pepper
1 onion
10 stuffed olives
14 fl oz (4 dl) tomato
 juice

Mix together the chili powder, cloves, caraway, pepper and salt, and rub both the inside and the outside of the chicken with the mixture. Save about a teaspoon of the spice mixture for the vegetables.

Dice the ham and chop the parsley. Add one pressed garlic clove and use the mixture to stuff the chicken. Place the chicken in a greased casserole and brush with the melted margarine.

Cut the green pepper into strips and chop the onion. Stir in the other pressed clove of garlic and the olives. Spread the vegetables around the chicken and sprinkle with the rest of the spice mixture. Pour the tomato juice over the vegetables and place the casserole in a very moderate oven, 350°F or Gas No 3 (175°C), for about one hour, basting occasionally. Serve with brown rice or a home-made bread.

Chicken Curry

2½ lb (1.1 kg) chicken
high-polyunsaturated
 margarine
salt and pepper
4 tsp curry powder
8-10 button onions
1 tbsp soy sauce
pinch cayenne pepper
 (optional)
1-2 apples
2 stalks celery

Joint the chicken and remove the skin. Brown the chicken pieces in a little margarine in a heavy saucepan. Add salt and pepper and sprinkle over the curry powder. Peel the onions and add to the pan. Pour on enough water to cover the chicken and onions. Add the soy sauce, and cayenne pepper if desired. Simmer for about an hour.

During this time, peel, core and cut the apples into small pieces. Slice the celery stalks. Sauté the apples and celery and add to the pan about 15 minutes before the end of the cooking time.

Serve with brown rice and a good salad.

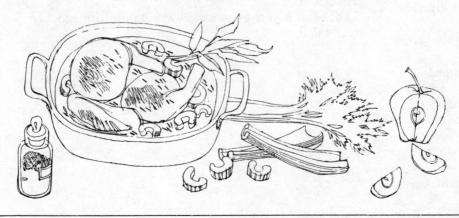

Indian Chicken with Spicy Rice

1 chicken about 2½ lb
(1.1 kg)
1 onion
2 tbsp polyunsaturated
oil
½ tsb coriander
¼ tsp caraway seed
¼ tsp black pepper
¼ tsp ginger
2 bay leaves
1 tsp salt
2 cloves garlic
9 fl oz (2.6 dl) water

SPICY RICE
14 fl oz (3.9 dl) water
½ tsp salt
1 tbsp polyunsaturated
oil
6 oz (170 g) long grain
rice
3 cardamom seeds
3 cloves
¼ tsp aniseed
1 cinnamon stick
½ packet saffron
3½ fl oz (1 dl)
skimmed milk
10 almonds
10-15 raisins

Joint the chicken and remove the skin. Place the peeled and chopped onion in a thick-bottomed saucepan and sauté in the oil until transparent. Add the spices, bay leaves, salt and pressed garlic and fry with the onion for a minute or two. Add the water and simmer for 10 minutes.

Put the chicken in the sauce, cover and continue to cook for about 25 minutes, by which time the sauce should be almost completely boiled off.

While the chicken is cooking, prepare the rice. Boil the water, salt and oil, add the rice and all the spices, cover and boil for about 20 minutes.

Place the rice and chicken in layers in a baking dish. Pour the milk over the rice and bake in a very hot oven, 500°F or Gas No 9 (260°C), for 15 minutes.

Scald and peel the almonds. Halve them and roast in a dry hot frying pan. Remove the chicken and rice from the oven. Garnish with raisins and roast almonds.

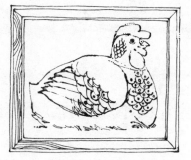

Chicken Tikka

1 chicken about 2½ lb
(1.1 kg)
10½ fl oz (3 dl) low
fat yogurt
½ tsp tumeric
1 tsp ginger
½ tsp black pepper
¼ tsp chili powder
mint
1 tsp salt
2 tbsp red wine
vinegar
1 lemon
4 cloves garlic

Joint the chicken and remove the skin. Mix the yogurt with all the spices, mint, salt, vinegar, lemon juice and pressed garlic. Marinate the chicken pieces in the mixture for 1½ hours.

Remove the chicken from the marinade and drain. Grill the pieces for 10-15 minutes, or place them in a roasting tin and bake in a very hot oven, 500°F or Gas No 9 (260°C) for 15 minutes, turning them once during this time.

Chicken in Curry Sauce

1 chicken about 3 lb
(1.3 kg)
1 carrot
1 leek
1 bay leaf
salt
10 black peppercorns

CURRY SAUCE
1-2 tsp curry powder
1 tbsp high-
polyunsaturated
margarine
10½ fl oz (3 dl)
chicken stock
3½ fl oz (1 dl)
skimmed milk
4 tbsp flour

Boil the chicken together with the carrot, leek, bay leaf, salt and peppercorns for about an hour. Fry the curry powder in the margarine. Add the chicken stock and the skimmed milk. Thicken the sauce with the flour stirred into a little water. Simmer for about 5 minutes.

Serve the chicken with brown rice and a green salad.

Any left-overs can be put back in the cooking liquid and used to make a good soup.

Benachin
Gambian National Dish

1 chicken about 2½ lb
(1.1 kg)
2 onions
2 tbsp polyunsaturated
oil
½ tbsp chili powder
1 tbsp paprika powder
2 14-oz (397-g) cans
tomatoes
1 tsp salt
12 fl oz (3.4 dl) water
1 marrow
2 avocados
2 small green sweet
peppers
1 small red sweet
pepper
1 small yellow sweet
pepper
6 oz (170 g) long
grain rice

Cut the chicken into pieces and remove the skin. Chop the onions and sauté them in the oil until they are transparent. Stir in the chili and paprika powders. Put the chicken pieces into the pan with the onions and spices and turn them until they are evenly covered with spices. Chop the tomatoes and add them to the pan with the tomato juice and water. Cover and simmer for about 15 minutes. Slice the marrow and cut each slice into 2 or 4 pieces. Peel and dice the avocados. Remove the seeds from the peppers and cut the flesh into strips. Measure out 14 fl oz (4 dl) of cooking liquid from the pan and use this to boil the rice over a low heat for 20 minutes. Stir the chopped vegetables (saving some for garnishing) into the pan with the chicken and allow to simmer for a further 5 minutes. Then turn the heat down very low so that it just keeps hot while the rice is cooking. Mix the contents of the pan into the rice. Place the chicken, rice and vegetable mixture on a serving dish and garnish with the raw vegetables.

Catalonian Chicken

1 chicken about 2½ lb
  (1.1 kg)
high-polyunsaturated
  margarine
salt and pepper
8 button onions
1 carrot
2 14-oz (397-g) cans
  tomatoes
1 bay leaf
½ tsp sweet basil
3½ fl oz (1 dl) water
1 green sweet pepper
chopped parsley

Joint the chicken and remove the skin. Brown the joints in a little margarine in a large heavy saucepan. Add salt and pepper. Peel the onions, slice the carrot and add to the pan. Pour in the tomatoes, add the bay leaf and sweet basil. Pour in the water and stir together. Cover and allow to simmer for about an hour. Dice the green pepper and add to the pan; sprinkle over the parsley just before serving. Serve with brown rice or boiled potatoes.

Chicken with Mushrooms and Almonds

1 chicken about 3 lb
  (1.4 kg)
1 tbsp polyunsaturated
  oil
salt and pepper
1 portion Stewed
  Mushrooms (see
  p. 62)
2-3 tbsp flaked
  almonds

Joint the chicken and remove the skin. Place the joints in a greased casserole and brush with the oil. Salt and pepper. Put the casserole in a moderately hot oven, 400°F or Gas No 5 (200°C). After 40 minutes remove the casserole from the oven and pour over the stewed mushrooms. Sprinkle each piece of chicken with the flaked almonds and return to the oven for a further 25 minutes. Serve with a crisp salad.

Enchiladas Tlaloc

8 tortillas (see
  p.124)
1 grilled chicken
2 8-oz (226-g) packets
  frozen broccoli
½ portion White
  Sauce
  (see p. 62)
low fat yogurt
low fat cottage cheese
tabasco

Place 4 tortillas in a greased oven dish. Remove the skin and bones from the chicken and dice the flesh. Divide the chicken flesh between the tortillas and cover with thawed broccoli. Top the chicken and broccoli with the remaining 4 tortillas. Mix together equal amounts of white sauce and low fat yogurt, and pour the mixture over the tortillas. Sprinkle with a few spoonsful of low fat cottage cheese and place a dash of tabasco on each tortilla.

Bake in a moderately hot oven, 400°F or Gas No 6 (200°C), for about 20 minutes.

This recipe may be varied by using grilled or boiled veal instead of chicken, or spinach instead of broccoli.

Chicken with Asparagus and Pimento

1 boiling chicken
2 onions
3 cloves
1 carrot
1 bay leaf
1-2 sprigs parsley
10 peppercorns
2 tsp salt

SAUCE
1 tbsp high-
    polyunsaturated
    margarine
2 tbsp flour
½ pint (2.8 dl)
    chicken stock
2 fl oz skimmed milk
1 10½-oz (300-g) can
    asparagus
3 whole canned
    pimentos

Remove all visible fat from the chicken and place it in a saucepan. Pour over sufficient water to cover, bring to the boil and skim. Peel the onions and insert the cloves. Scrub the carrot and cut into thin slices. Add the vegetables, bay leaf, parsley sprigs, peppercorns and salt to the chicken, and boil for about 2 hours or until the chicken is tender. Lift the chicken from the stock, let the stock cool, and skim as much fat from the surface as possible.

Remove the skin and bones from the chicken and dice the flesh. Take one pint of the stock and boil it down to ½ pint to concentrate the flavour.

Melt the margarine, stir in the flour and cook gently for a minute or two. Stir in the ½ pint chicken stock, skimmed milk and water from the asparagus. Allow to simmer for a few minutes. Cut the pimentos into thin strips and stir into the sauce together with the asparagus and the chicken meat, and bring to the boil. Serve immediately with boiled rice.

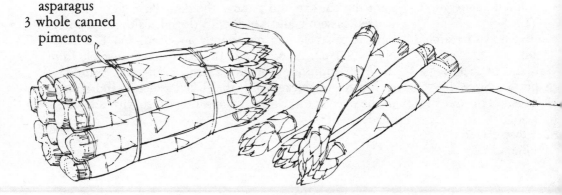

Chicken Supreme

1 boiled or grilled
    chicken about
    2½ lb (1.1 kg)
1 onion
8 oz (226 g)
    mushrooms
1 5-oz (142-g) can peas
1 portion White Sauce
    (see p. 62)
1½ tsp French
    mustard (Dijon)
2-3 tbsp sherry

Remove the skin from the chicken. Lift the flesh from the bones and dice it. Peel and chop the onion. Clean and slice the mushrooms.

Make one portion of white sauce, but with a thicker consistency than usual. Add the mustard and sherry.

Place the chicken flesh, onion, mushrooms and drained peas in a casserole. Pour over the sauce and stir together. Cover and place the casserole in a moderately hot oven, 400°F for Gas No 5 (200°C), for 40 minutes.

Chicken Florentine

1 lb (454 g) fresh
   spinach
   or
2 8-oz (226-g) packets
   frozen spinach
1 grilled or boiled
   chicken
salt and pepper
ground nutmeg
4 oz (113 g) low fat
   cottage cheese
1 lemon
3 egg whites

Rinse the spinach and boil it in lightly salted water for 5 minutes. Pour into a strainer, drain and then press with a spoon to get all the water out. (Frozen spinach should be prepared according to the instructions on the packet.)

Skin the chicken and remove the flesh from the bones. Dice the chicken meat. Make a bed of spinach at the bottom of a greased baking dish, season with salt and pepper and grate a little nutmeg over it. Arrange the pieces of chicken in a layer over the spinach. Mix the cottage cheese with the grated peel of half a lemon and 1 tbsp lemon juice. Add salt and pepper to taste.

Beat the egg whites until stiff and fold in the cottage cheese mixture. Cover the chicken with the foamy batter and bake in a very hot oven, 500°F or Gas No 9 (260°C), until the batter is a beautiful brown, about 5-10 minutes.

Chicken à Porto

4 chicken breasts
   about 2 lb (9 hg)
salt and pepper
¼ tsp sweet basil
4 slices lemon
7 fl oz (2 dl) port wine
2 7½-oz (213-g)
   cans mushrooms

Place the four chicken breasts on large sheet of aluminium foil. Season with salt, pepper and sweet basil. Put a slice of lemon on each chicken breast. Pull the aluminium foil together to make an airtight packet. Bake in a moderately hot oven, 400°F or Gas No 5 (200°C), for 40 minutes.

Turkey in Wine

10-12 PERSONS
1 10-lb (4.5-kg) turkey
salt
10 onions
3½ pints (2 l) chicken
   stock
1¾ pints (1 l) water
17 fl oz (5 dl) dry
   vermouth
2 tbsp high-
   polyunsaturated
   margarine
2 tbsp flour
1-2 tbsp soy sauce

Salt the inside of the turkey and tie up the legs. Peel the onions and boil with the neck, heart and gizzard in the stock and water for 35 minutes. Strain the stock and mix it with the vermouth, adding salt if necessary. Place the turkey in the wine and stock mixture and boil slowly for 1-1½ hours or until the flesh is tender. Remove the bird and keep hot. Skim the fat floating on the surface of the stock, and boil until only about 1¾ pints (1 l) remain.

Melt the margarine in a saucepan, stir in the flour and cook gently for a few minutes. Stir into the stock mixture and season with the soy sauce. Carve the turkey, and place the meat on a serving platter. Pour over a little of the sauce.

Serve with rice, the rest of the sauce, asparagus and a crisp salad.

Larry's Stuffed Turkey

ABOUT 10 PERSONS
1 8-lb (3.6-kg) turkey
polyunsaturated oil
salt and pepper
2 apples
2 onions
3 stalks celery
7 oz (198 g) chopped
   walnuts
5 oz (141 g)
   breadcrumbs
7 fl oz (2 dl) sherry

Brush the turkey with oil, and salt and pepper the outside. Peel and chop the apples and onions, and slice the celery. Place the chopped vegetables and apples in a large bowl and add the walnuts, breadcrumbs and sherry. Salt and pepper to taste, mix well and stuff the turkey with the mixture.

Place the turkey on a grid over a roasting pan, with water in the pan to catch the drips.

Bake for 2½ hours in a very moderate oven, 350°F or Gas No 3 (175°C), basting occasionally.

Serve with mashed potatoes, petits pois and a salad.

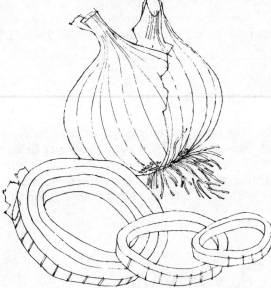

Meat

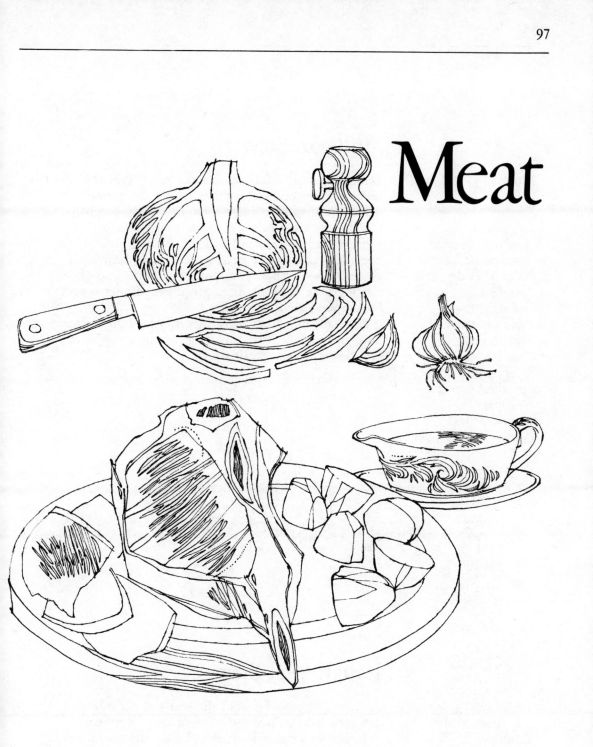

Mulligan Stew

1 lb (454 g) lean beef
1 large onion
2 carrots
1 tbsp high-
   polyunsaturated
   margarine
3½ fl oz (1 dl)
   white wine
1 14-oz (397-g)
   can tomatoes
2 cloves garlic
1 bay leaf
½ tsp thyme
a pinch of cayenne
   pepper
salt and pepper
1 green sweet pepper

Remove all visible fat and dice the meat. Peel and slice the onion and carrots, and fry them in the margarine until the onion is transparent. Place them in a large saucepan together with the meat. Add the wine, tomatoes and sufficient water to cover. Add the crushed garlic, herbs, cayenne pepper and seasoning. Cover and simmer for about 2 hours. About 5 minutes before the end of the cooking time, add the diced green pepper. Serve with boiled potatoes or brown rice.

Naturally any other vegetables may be used according to taste and time of year. Try using parsnips, swedes or cauliflower, to name just a few.

Italian Veal Stew

1½ lb (680 g) lean
   boneless veal
1 onion
1 clove garlic
1 tbsp
   polyunsaturated
   oil
salt and pepper
¼ tsp sage
5½ fl oz (1.6 dl)
   tomato juice
3½ fl oz (1 dl)
   white wine

Remove all visible fat from the veal and cut it into 1½-inch cubes. Place the cubes of meat in a heavy saucepan or a casserole. Peel and chop the onion and garlic, and fry them in a little oil until the onion is transparent. Season with salt and pepper and sprinkle in the sage. Stir in the tomato juice and wine and allow to simmer for a while. Pour the sauce over the meat and cover with a lid or aluminium foil. Put the meat and sauce in a hot oven, 430°F or Gas No 6-7 (225°C), for ¾-1 hour, or until the meat is tender.

Serve with noodles and boiled carrots and onions.

Baked Pork Chops

4 large pork chops
   or
8 lamb chops
salt and pepper
2 onions
polyunsaturated
   margarine
10 potatoes
1 clove garlic
2 bay leaves
½ tsp thyme
10½ fl oz (3 dl)
   beef stock
3 tbsp concentrated
   tomato purée

Season the chops with salt and pepper and grill them for 2 minutes on each side. Peel and slice the onions and fry them slowly in a little margarine. Peel the potatoes and cut in thin slices.

Rub a casserole with the juice of the crushed garlic. Grease it and make a bed of the potato slices. Cover the potatoes with the onions, sprinkle with the herbs and top with the chops. Bring the beef stock to the boil and stir the tomato purée into it. Pour this mixture over the chops. There should be sufficient liquid to cover the potatoes.

Bake in a hot oven, 430°F or Gas No 6-7 (225°C), for about 30 minutes.

Veal Tarragon

1¼ lb (5.7 hg) lean
   boneless veal
2 carrots
2 onions
1 bay leaf
8 peppercorns
2 tbsp flour
3½ fl oz (1 dl)
   skimmed milk
2 tbsp high-
   polyunsaturated
   margarine
1 egg yolk
¼ - ½ tsp tarragon
salt and pepper
8 oz (226 g)
   mushrooms
1 bunch parsley

Remove all visible fat from the veal and cut it into cubes. Put the meat into a saucepan and pour on sufficient water to cover. Bring to the boil and skim.

Peel the carrots and onions and cut them into pieces. Add to the saucepan along with the spices. Allow to simmer for about an hour or until the meat is tender.

Strain the meat stock into a second saucepan. Stir the flour into a little of the milk. Bring the meat stock to the boil, and add the diluted flour and 1 tbsp of margarine.

Beat the egg yolk in a bowl with a little of the milk. Add a few spoonsful of the stock while beating, and then pour the egg and meat stock into the sauce. Bring the sauce to the boil, stirring constantly. Remove from the heat and dilute with the rest of the milk. Season with the tarragon, salt and pepper.

Rinse and clean the mushrooms and sauté them in the remaining margarine. Fold the meat and mushrooms into the sauce and allow to simmer for 5 minutes. Sprinkle with plenty of chopped parsley and serve with boiled rice.

Wine Marinated Pork Roast

2 lb (9 hg) roasting
  joint of pork
2 tbsp melted high-
  polyunsaturated
  margarine
¼ tsp black pepper
¼ tsp ground cloves
½ tsp thyme
½ tsp salt

MARINADE

½ pint (2.8 dl)
  dry white wine
2 tbsp concentrated
  tomato purée
3 tbsp red wine
  vinegar
1 tbsp soy sauce
2 onions
2 carrots
2 stalks celery
1 bunch parsley

Mix the liquid ingredients for the marinade. Peel and slice the onion, slice the carrot and celery and chop the parsley. Mix the spices and rub into the roast. Place the meat in a large bowl, cover with the chopped vegetables, and pour over the marinade. Cover and allow to stand in a cool place for 2 to 12 hours. Remove the joint and place it on a grid set over a roasting pan. Brush with the margarine and season. Cook in a very moderate oven, 350°F or Gas No 3 (175°C), for 25 minutes.

Strain the marinade. Place the vegetables in a baking dish, pour on about 3½ fl oz (1 dl) of the marinade, and put the dish in the oven along with the roast. Pour the rest of the marinade over the roast and cook for a further 50 minutes, basting occasionally.

Allow the roast to rest for about 15 minutes before carving.

Roast Lamb with Herbs

2 lb (9 hg) lean
  roasting
  joint of lamb
salt and pepper
2-3 tbsp high-
  polyunsaturated
  margarine
1 small onion
¾ tsp chervil
¾ tsp sage
¾ tsp thyme

Rub the lamb with salt and pepper. Make a paste of the margarine, finely chopped onion and herbs, and spread the paste evenly over the lamb.

Place on a grid over a roasting pan and cook in a very moderate oven, 350°F or Gas No 3 (175°C), for about an hour. If the meat seems to be getting too dark, cover with aluminium foil. Allow the roast to rest for about 15 minutes before carving.

Other good spices for lamb prepared in this way are sage and sweet basil, or rosemary.

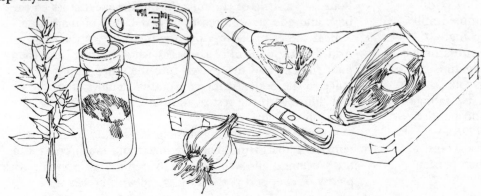

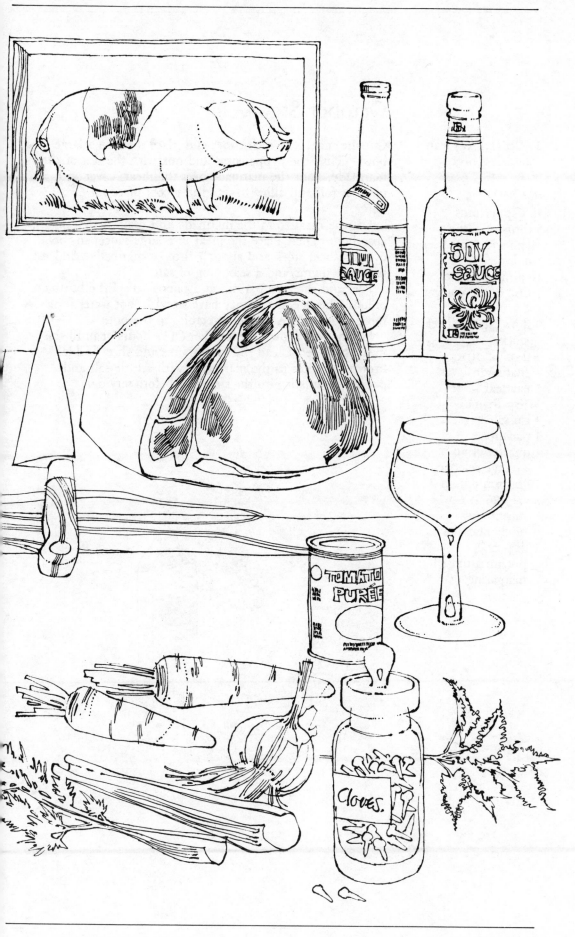

October Stew

2 ½ lb (1.1 kg) lean
boneless beef

MARINADE
10 peppercorns
5 corns of allspice
½ pint (2.8 dl) beer
1 onion
10 juniper berries
1 tbsp apple vinegar

9 fl oz (2.5 dl) beef
stock
7 fl oz (2 dl)
marinade
1 bay leaf
¼ tsp thyme
1 tsp salt
1 parsnip
1 quarter of an
average celeriac
10 button onions
8 oz (226 g)
mushrooms
or chantarelles
1 tbsp high-
polyunsaturated
margarine

Cut the meat in 1-inch cubes and place them in a large
bowl. Crush the peppercorns and mix with the rest of the
marinade. Pour the marinade over the meat, cover with a
plate or foil and allow to stand in a cool place for 6 to 12
hours.

Lift the meat from the marinade and drain it well on
absorbent paper. Place the meat in a large saucepan, pour
over the beef stock and about 7 fl oz of marinade. Add the
bay leaf, thyme and a seasoning of salt.

Peel and slice the parsnip and celeriac. Peel the button
onions (this is easier if they have stood in hot water for a
minute or two). Add the vegetables to the pot.

Simmer on a low heat for about 1½ hours or until the
meat is tender. Clean the mushrooms and slice thickly,
brown the slices in the margarine with a little salt and
pepper, then stir into the stew just before serving.

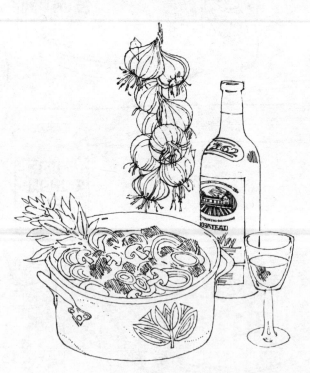

American Tagliatelle

1 lb (454 g) minced
  beef
1 onion
high-
  polyunsaturated
  margarine
tagliatelle
1 5-oz (140-g) can
  concentrated tomato
  purée
5 ½ fl oz (1.6 dl) water
2 cloves garlic
1 tsp oregano
1 tsp chili powder
a few drops tabasco
2 8-oz (226-g) packets
  frozen broccoli
1 portion White Sauce
  (*see* p. 62)
ground nutmeg
1 11½-oz (326-g) can
  sweet corn

Buy lean beef. Trim away any fat and pass through a mincer. Peel and chop the onion and fry it together with the minced beef in a little margarine. Put it aside.

Use less tagliatelle than normal for four people and boil it until almost cooked.

Mix together the tomato purée, water, pressed garlic, oregano, chili powder and tabasco to make a tomato sauce. Cook the broccoli according to the instructions on the packet.

Make one portion of white sauce seasoned with nutmeg. Drain the pasta well and place it in the bottom of a greased casserole. Next make a layer of the meat and onion, and pour the tomato sauce over this. Then make a layer of sweet corn and top it with the broccoli. Pour the white sauce over the broccoli. Put the casserole in a very hot oven, 475°F or Gas No 8 (250°C), for about 30 minutes or until the white sauce has an attractive colour.

Serve with a crisp fresh salad.

Pork and Cabbage

1 lb (454 g) lean pork
1 cabbage about
  2 lb (9 hg)
2-3 onions
salt and pepper
1 tsp sweet basil
water or beef stock

Remove all visible fat and cut the meat into thin slices. Chop the cabbage and onions. Arrange the meat, cabbage, onions and spices in layers in a heavy saucepan. Pour on sufficient water or stock to cover one-third of the contents of the pan. Cover with a lid and simmer for about 45 minutes. Serve with boiled potatoes.

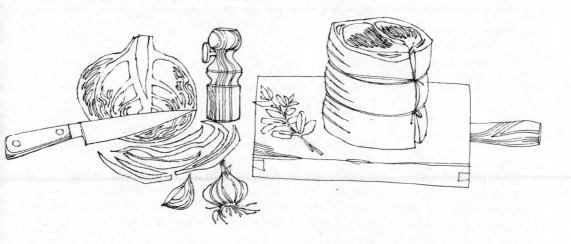

Roast Beef with Garlic

ABOUT 10 PERSONS

4½ lb (2 kg) boned
   and rolled roasting
   joint of beef
fresh garlic
salt and pepper

Remove all visible fat. Cut small holes in the meat, about 1½ inches deep and equidistant from each other. Insert whole or half cloves of garlic in each hole. Dust with salt and pepper. Place the roast on a grid set over a roasting pan and bake in a hot oven, 425°F or Gas No 6-7 (225°C), for about 1 to 1½ hours, depending on the degree of rareness preferred.

Serve with Potato Casserole (*see* p. 75) or baked potatoes.

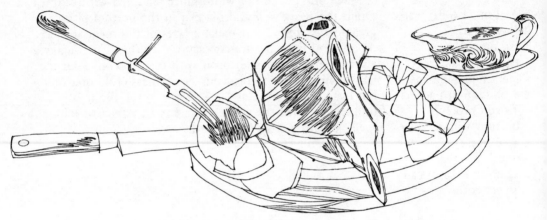

Pork Tenderloin with Stewed Mushrooms

1 lb (454 g) tenderloin
   of pork
salt and pepper
1 portion Stewed
   Mushrooms (*see*
   p. 62)
4 tomatoes
1 tbsp melted high-
   polyunsaturated
   margarine
½ tsp oregano

Remove all visible fat from the tenderloin, season with salt and pepper and place in a greased baking dish. Pour over the stewed mushrooms. Rinse and halve the tomatoes, place them in the dish around the meat. Brush the tomatoes with the melted margarine, and sprinkle with a little oregano. Bake in a moderately hot oven, 400°F or Gas No 5 (200°C), for about 40 minutes.

Beef Tartar

PER PERSON

about 6 oz (170 g)
   lean minced beef
capers
chopped onion
chopped beetroots

Buy lean beef, remove all visible fat, and pass through a mincer.

Shape the beef mince into a patty. Garnish with 3 onion rings filled with capers, chopped onion and beets. The capers, onion, and beets can also be mixed into the minced meat if desired. Serve with Tomato and Mushroom Salad (*see* p.54).

Spiced Surprise

4 large thin slices
   topside of beef
salt and pepper
1 onion
2 tbsp grated
   horseradish
1 tbsp French
   mustard (Dijon)
1 tbsp capers
1 tbsp polyunsaturated
   oil
1 tbsp soy sauce

Beat the meat to flatten it, and salt and pepper on one side. Chop the onion very finely and mix it with the horseradish, mustard and capers. Divide the mixture between the meat slices on the seasoned side and fold the meat over the filling, fastening it with a toothpick. Mix the oil and soy sauce and brush over the meat. Grill the meat about 3 minutes on each side, turning carefully so as not to spill the filling. Serve with a baked potato and a crisp salad.

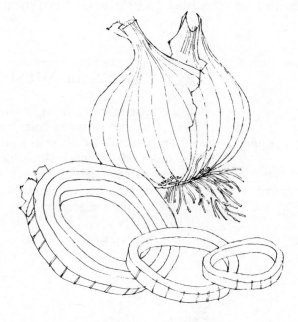

Enchiladas de Cochinita

about 1 lb (454 g)
   lean pork
2 onions
polyunsaturated
   margarine
1 tsp nutmeg
salt and pepper
8 tortillas
   (*see* p. 124)
7 fl oz (2 dl) Red
   Chili Sauce (*see*
   p. 64)
2-3 tbsp (low fat)
   cottage cheese

Remove all visible fat from the meat and cut it into ¼-inch cubes. Quarter and slice one of the onions. Fry the meat and sliced onion in a little margarine and season with the nutmeg, salt and pepper.

Dip one tortilla in the chili sauce until soft and roll it round a heaped spoonful of the meat and onion mixture. Do likewise with the other tortillas and place them in a greased baking dish. Chop the remaining onion and sprinkle over the tortilla rolls. Pour over the remaining sauce and sprinkle over the cottage cheese.

Bake in a moderately hot oven, 400°F or Gas No 5 (200°C), until thoroughly hot, about 15 minutes.

Psito me Patates

8-10 potatoes
1 14-oz (397-g) can
    tomatoes
1 bunch parsley
1-2 tsp salt
1 tsp black pepper
4-6 slices lean pork
soy sauce
4 tbsp
    polyunsaturated oil

Peel and quarter the potatoes, and place them in the bottom of a greased baking dish. Pour over the tinned tomatoes, crushing them first, and sprinkle over the chopped parsley. Season with salt and pepper. Arrange the pork slices on the top, season with salt and pepper, and brush them with a little soy sauce. Drip the oil over the top and bake in a very hot oven, 500°F or Gas No 9 (260°C), for 15 minutes; then lower the temperature to very moderate, 350°F or Gas No 3 (175°C), and bake for a further 25-30 minutes. Turn the pork slices once during the cooking time.

Tagliatelle à la Westeaud

tagliatelle
4 tomatoes
1 green sweet pepper
1 leek
2 tbsp
    polyunsaturated oil
12 oz (340 g) lean
    boiled ham
15-20 olives
salt and pepper

Boil the tagliatelle according to the instructions on the packet. Dice the tomatoes and green pepper, and slice the leek. Fry them all lightly in the oil, but not enough to make them soft. Remove all visible fat from the ham and cut into small squares.

When the noodles are almost ready, pour off the water and add the fried vegetables, ham and olives. Return the pan to a low heat and stir together until everything is nice and hot. Salt and pepper to taste.

Gothenburgers

1 lb (454 g) minced
    beef
2 tsp potato flour
2 tbsp cold water
2 drops tabasco
½ tsp Worcestershire
    sauce
¼ tsp garlic powder
salt and pepper
2 stalks celery
1 small onion
1 egg white
1 tbsp polyunsaturated
    oil
1 tbsp soy sauce

Mince the meat rather coarsely. Mix the potato flour with the water and add the meat and spices. Chop the celery and onion very finely, add them to the meat mixture and stir in the egg white. Add the polyunsaturated oil and soy sauce and mix well.

Shape the meat into 4 large patties and brush with the soy and oil mixture. Grill the patties 2-3 minutes on each side.

Baked Ham with Broccoli and Mushrooms

1 lb (454 g) broccoli
1 lb (454 g) sliced
   lean boiled ham
1 portion
   Stewed Mushrooms
   (*see* p. 62)

Boil the broccoli in lightly salted water for 6-8 minutes. Then place it in a greased baking dish and cover with a layer of ham slices. Over this pour the stewed mushrooms. Bake in a very hot oven, 475°F or Gas No 8 (250°C) for about 20 minutes.

Served with hot Poppy Rolls (*see* p.122) and a salad, this is a delicious lunch or supper.

The recipe may be varied by exchanging the ham for pieces of chicken or veal.

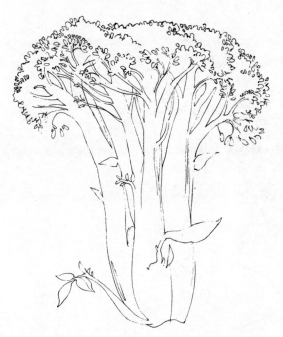

Desserts

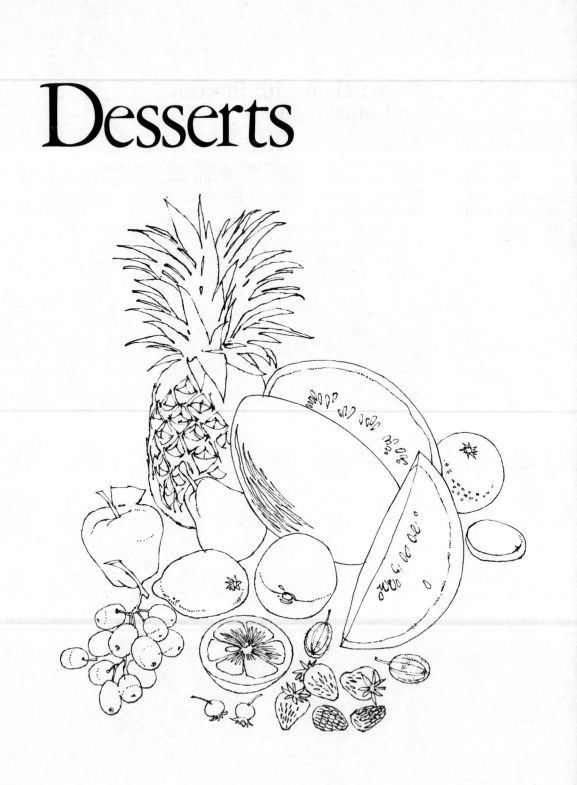

Apple Pie

6-8 PERSONS

CRUST
10 oz (284 g) flour
3 tbsp chopped
    almonds
4½ fl oz (1.25 dl)
    polyunsaturated oil
5 tbsp ice-cold water

FILLING
2 lb (9 hg) apples
3-4 tbsp sugar
½ tbsp cinnamon
3 tbsp raisins

Mix the flour and almonds in a large bowl. Stir the oil and water together and pour the mixture over the flour. Mix to a dough and knead until smooth. Divide the dough into two parts, one larger than the other. Roll out the larger part to a circle large enough to cover an 8½-inch pie-dish. Fit carefully into the dish so that bottom and sides are completely covered. Roll out the remaining dough ready for the top.

Peel, core and quarter the apples. Cut the quarters into slices, and simmer in as little water as possible for about 3-4 minutes. Remove the apples, allow them to drain, and spread them evenly over the pastry base in the pie-dish. Sprinkle over the sugar, cinnamon and raisins, and cover with the pastry top. Pinch the edges of the top and bottom together to seal, and puncture the top with a fork to allow the steam to escape. Trim the edges of the pie neatly to give an attractive appearance.

Bake in a moderately hot oven, 400°F or Gas No 5 (200°C), for 45-50 minutes.

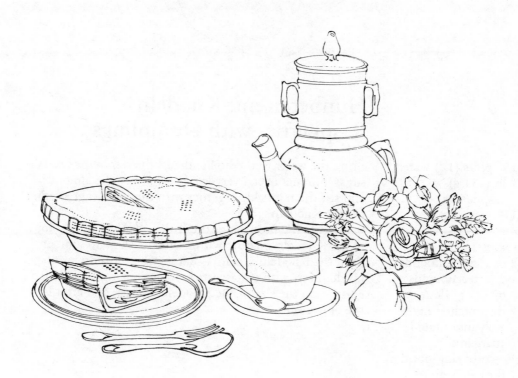

Greek Plums

8 large ripe plums
strong hot tea
4 tbsp honey
4 tbsp chopped
  walnuts

Halve the plums and remove the stones. Place the plums in a bowl, pour over sufficient tea to cover them, and allow to steep for about an hour before removing from the tea and peeling them. Heat the honey in a saucepan, add the plums and heat them thoroughly. Place in dessert bowls, pour over the honey and sprinkle with nuts. Serve with low fat yogurt, if desired.

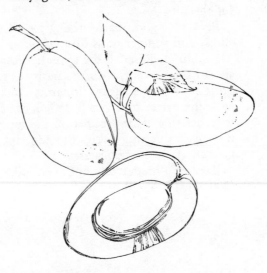

Himberen mit Knödeln
Raspberries with Dumplings

1¾ pints (1 l) water
1 lb (454 g)
  raspberries
1½ tbsp sugar

KNÖDELN
2 oz (56 g) almonds
1-2 bitter almonds
3 oz (85 g) flour
2 tbsp melted high-
  polyunsaturated
  margarine
½ tsp baking powder
2 fl oz (0.5 dl)
  skimmed milk
¼ tsp salt

Bring the water to the boil and add the raspberries and sugar. Simmer over a very low heat. Mince the almonds and stir them quickly together with the other ingredients for the Knödeln.

  Increase the heat under the fruit and add a few dollops of the Knödeln mixture with a spoon. Allow to simmer until the Knödeln is ready, that is, when it is dry on the inside. (Test with a matchstick.) The cooking time depends entirely on the size of the Knödeln, so trial and error is the only guide.

Raspberry Pears

4 pears
7 fl oz (2 dl) white
  wine
8 oz (226 g) fresh
  raspberries
1 tbsp sugar

Peel, core and quarter the pears. Bring the wine to the boil, add the pears and allow to simmer for about 5 minutes or until they are almost soft. Remove the pears and cool.

Place the raspberries in a bowl and sprinkle with the sugar. Leave to stand for several hours. Press the berries through a sieve, then pour the raspberry purée over the pears and serve.

Grapefruit Dessert

1 grapefruit
2 oz (56 g) shelled
  walnuts
1 lb (454 g)
  raspberries
8 oz (226 g) low fat
  cottage cheese

Peel and chop the grapefruit. Chop the nuts. Mix together the grapefruit flesh, nuts and raspberries. Place a layer of cottage cheese in the base of 4 dessert bowls and divide the fruit mixture between them. Serve chilled.

Banana Flambé

4 bananas
high-polyunsaturated
  margarine
2 tbsp brandy
6 tbsp flaked almonds
8 oz (226 g) low fat
  cottage cheese

Peel the bananas and fry them in margarine over a low heat for about 5 minutes. Pour on the brandy and ignite. Allow to burn for about a minute before smothering the fire with the lid of the frying pan. Toast the almonds in a dry frying pan. Place each banana on a dessert plate and divide the cottage cheese among the plates. Garnish with the almonds.

Prune Marmalade

8 oz (226 g) stoned
  prunes
5 ½ fl oz (1.5 dl) water
1 tsp grated lemon
  peel
3 ½ oz (100 g)
  almonds
2 tbsp sugar
1 tsp ginger

Mix the prunes, water and lemon peel in a pan and
simmer for 35 minutes. Chop the almonds. Remove the
pan from the heat and mash the prunes with a spoon. Stir
in the sugar, chopped almonds and ginger.

This marmalade should be kept in the refrigerator.

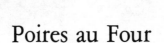

Poires au Four

4 large ripe pears
1 lemon
3 tbsp sugar
3 tbsp melted high-
  polyunsaturated
  margarine

Peel and halve the pears and brush them with lemon juice
to prevent discoloration. Place the pear halves in a greased
baking dish. Grate the peel of half a well washed lemon
and mix with the sugar. Divide this mixture over the pears
and pour on the melted margarine.

Bake in a very hot oven, 500°F or Gas No 9 (260°C), for
10 minutes. Baste the pears once during the cooking time.
Serve hot with cold low fat cottage cheese.

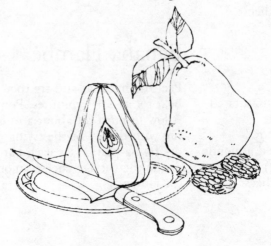

Fruit-filled Pineapple

ABOUT 6 PERSONS
1 pineapple about
   3¼ lb (1.5 kg)
2-3 satsumas
8 oz (226 g) black
   grapes

Cut the top off the pineapple and scoop out the inside flesh. Cut the flesh into small cubes. Peel and section the satsumas. Rinse the grapes, cut them in two and remove the seeds.

Take a slice from the base of the pineapple so that it will stand upright. Place the pineapple shell on a serving plate and fill with a mixture of the satsuma sections, grape halves and pineapple cubes. Pour all the juice into the shell. Replace the top of the pineapple and place the remaining fruit mixture around the shell. Serve chilled.

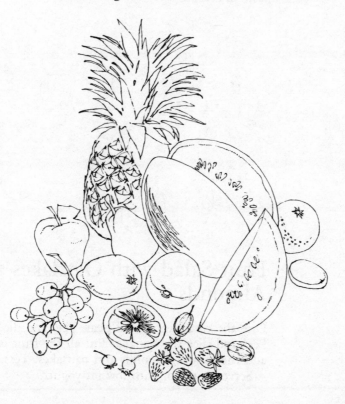

Baked Apples

4-6 apples
2 oz (56 g) almonds
3 tbsp raisins
3-4 tbsp sweet sherry
2 tbsp melted high-
   polyunsaturated
   margarine

Wash and core the apples. Chop and mix together the almonds and raisins. Place the apples in a greased baking dish and stuff them with the almond and raisin mixture. Pour in enough sherry to cover the bottom of the dish, and pour the melted margarine over the apples.

Bake in a very moderate oven, 350°F or Gas No 3 (175°C), for 20-30 minutes or until the apples are soft. The cooking time can vary considerably depending on the size and type of apples.

Fruit in Jelly

6 PERSONS
4-5 oranges
8 oz (226 g) grapes
3 tsp gelatine powder
1 pt (5.6 dl) orange
  juice

Peel the oranges and slice them in attractive cross-sections. Slice the grapes in two and remove the seeds. Place the fruit on one large serving plate or divide between individual dessert bowls.

Dissolve the gelatine in a little boiling water and dilute it with the orange juice. Pour this solution over the fruit and put in a cool place to set.

Naturally this can be varied with other fruit, for example pineapple and keewee, or peaches and limes, according to taste or season.

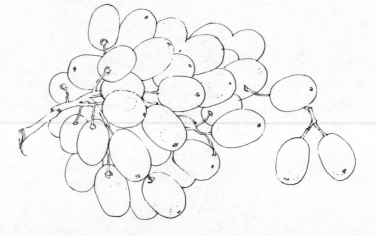

Fruit Salad with Oatflakes and Almonds

1 apple
1 pear
2 oranges
1 banana
2 tbsp raisins
2 tbsp chopped
  almonds
3 tbsp oatflakes

Dice the cored apple and pear. Peel and dice the oranges. Peel and slice the banana. Put all the fruit into a bowl and add the raisins, almonds and oatflakes. Toss.

Serve as it is or with low fat yogurt.

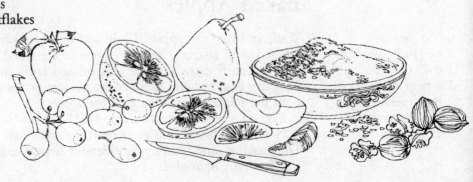

Drinks

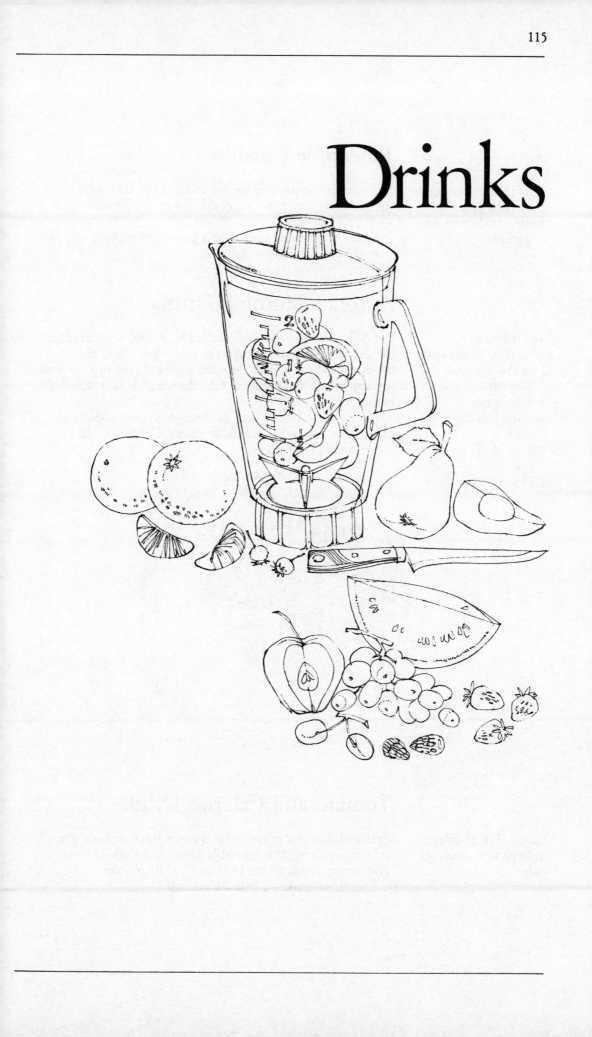

Pineapple Crush

8 oz (226 g) pineapple
8 oz (226 g) melon
fresh strawberries for
    garnish

Peel the pineapple and melon and cut the flesh into
pieces. Press through a vegetable juicer. This yields about
14 fl oz (4 dl) juice.

Pour the foaming juice into a glass over crushed ice, and
garnish with strawberry halves.

Aurora's Morning Drink

ABOUT 5 PERSONS
17½ fl oz (5 dl) water
2 oz (56 g) dried
    rose hips
1 tbsp honey
½ pint (2.8 dl) apple
    juice
7 fl oz (2 dl) grape
    juice
1 lemon

Bring the water to the boil and add the rose hips. Simmer
for about 10 minutes. Strain the rose hips, stir in the
honey and allow to cool. Mix the honeyed rose hip tea with
the apple and grape juices. Add the sliced lemon. Chill
before serving.

This drink is best if you can press your own apple and
grape juice through a vegetable juicer. Otherwise use
unsweetened fruit juices.

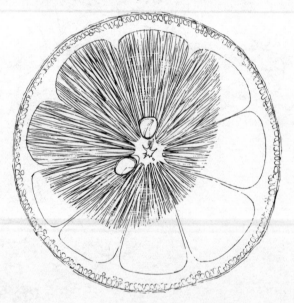

Tomato and Celeriac Drink

12 oz (340 g) celeriac
6 large ripe tomatoes
salt

Peel and dice the celeriac and quarter the tomatoes. Press
everything through a vegetable juicer. Add salt to taste.
This recipe yields about 18 fl oz (5.1 dl) of juice.

This drink makes a delicate aperitif.

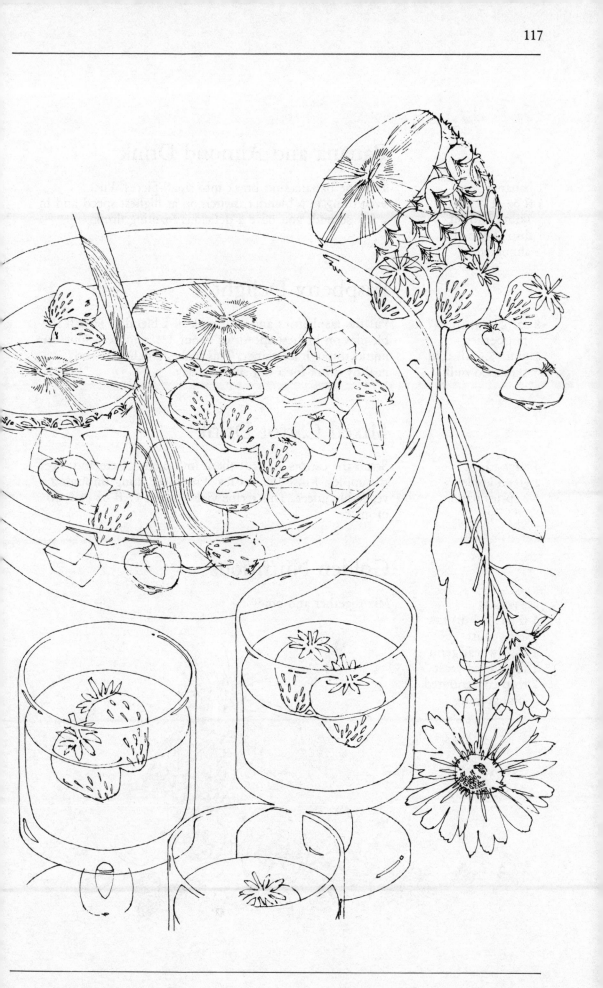

Banana and Almond Drink

1 banana
5 fl oz (1.4 dl)
  skimmed milk
1 tbsp chopped
  almonds

Peel the banana and break into small pieces. Put everything in a blender, switch on at highest speed and in a few seconds you have a delicious foaming drink.

Raspberry Delight

8 oz (226 g) fresh
  raspberries
1 pint (5.6 dl) cold
  skimmed milk

Put the raspberries and cold milk in a blender. Switch the blender on highest speed for about 1½ minutes. Pour the liquid through a strainer. This makes a delicious and healthy drink for a hot summer day.

Mixed Carrot Drink

4 large carrots
2 green apples
1-2 sprigs parsley

Scrub the carrots and cut them into pieces. Core and dice the apples. Rinse the parsley. Press everything through a vegetable juicer. This recipe yields about 17 fl oz (4.8 dl) of juice.

Golden Nutritious

PER PERSON
5 fl oz (1.4 dl) low
  fat yogurt
1 tbsp wheat germ
1 tbsp dried yeast
2 tbsp concentrated
  orange juice

Mix together and enjoy.

Bread

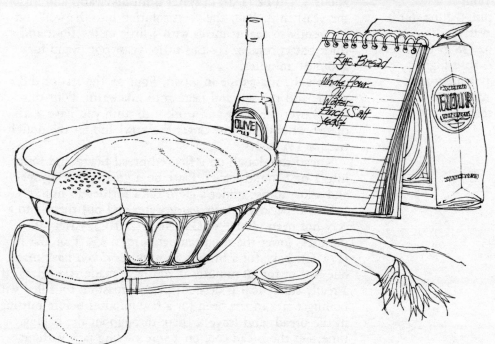

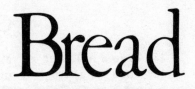

Country Bread

1½ lb (6.8 hg) flour
10½ oz (300 g) rye
flour
1 pint 5 fl oz (6 dl)
water
1 oz (28 g) fresh yeast
2½ tbsp high-
polyunsaturated
margarine
1 tbsp salt

Mix together the two types of flour in a large bowl, and make a well in the centre about the size of an egg. Heat about 3½ fl oz (1 dl) of water until lukewarm and dissolve the yeast in it. Pour the yeast solution into the well and stir gently so that it mixes with a little of the flour and a thick batter results. Let this little 'yeast pot' stand for about 30 minutes.

Melt the margarine in a pan. Pour on the rest of the water, add the salt and heat until lukewarm. Pour this liquid over the flour and work it in until you have a shiny dough without lumps. Cover the bowl and let the dough rise for 1½ hours.

Knead the dough on a floured bread board and form into 1 or 2 round loaves. Place on a greased baking sheet and allow to rise under a cloth for a further 15 minutes.

Brush the loaves with warm water and put them into a very hot oven, 500°F or Gas No 9 (260°C). After 10 minutes, lower the oven temperature to 350°F or Gas No 3 (175°C); bake for a further 50 minutes if you have made one loaf or for 30 minutes if you have made two loaves. If a really crusty loaf is desired, place a roasting tin filled with boiling water in the oven for a few minutes before putting in the bread, and leave it there throughout the baking time. Let the bread cool on a wire cooling rack without being covered with a cloth. This bread keeps very well and the crust can be kept at its best if the loaf is merely wrapped in a tea towel and placed with the cut surface down.

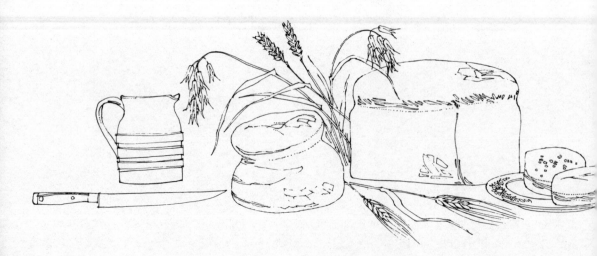

Rye Bread

2 oz (56 g) fresh yeast
18 fl oz (5.1 dl) water
2 tbsp
    polyunsaturated oil
¼ tbsp salt
about 17 oz (481 g)
    rye flour
about 13 oz (368 g)
    plain white flour

Dissolve the yeast in lukewarm water in a large mixing bowl. Add the oil and salt and stir together. Stir in the flours, adding the rye first, until you have a smooth, rather thick dough. Knead the dough on a floured bread board, then return to the bowl and let it rise for about 40 minutes.

Put the dough on the bread board and divide it into two equal halves. Knead each half and form it into a loaf. Place the loaves on a greased baking sheet and let them rise for another 40 minutes.

Bake the loaves in a very moderate oven, 300°F or Gas No 2 (150°C), for about 40-50 minutes.

Nut Cake

1 egg
3½ tbsp high-
    polyunsaturated
    margarine
3½ fl oz (1 dl) apple
    juice
1 tbsp honey
6 oz (170 g) plain
    white flour
2 tsp baking powder
2½ oz (71 g) chopped
    walnuts
2 oz (56 g) chopped
    raisins
3 egg whites

Beat the egg until foamy. Melt the margarine, pour in the apple juice and honey and heat until very hot but not boiling. Stir the hot liquids into the beaten egg. In another bowl mix the flour, baking powder, nuts and raisins. Add the dry ingredients to the egg and juice mixture and stir until a batter is formed. In another bowl beat the egg whites until really stiff, thick enough to turn the bowl upside-down without spilling. Gently and carefully, fold the egg whites into the batter. Pour the batter into a greased, floured cake tin and bake in a very moderate oven, 350°F or Gas No 3 (175°C) for 45-50 minutes.

Wholewheat Bread

2 oz (56 g) yeast
1 pt 6 fl oz (7.4 dl)
    water (room
    temperature)
10 oz (284 g)
    wholewheat flour
18 oz (5.1 hg) plain
    white flour
2 tsp salt
4 tbsp melted high-
    polyunsaturated
    margarine

Dissolve the yeast in the water, and add the wholewheat flour. This should result in a thick batter. Leave to stand for about an hour to give the yeast a chance to ferment. Stir down with a spoon and add the white flour, salt and melted margarine. Knead lightly on a floured board, shape into two loaves and place in bread pans. Allow to rise for about an hour and bake in a moderate oven, 375°F or Gas No 4 (200°C) for approximately 30 minutes. This bread is suitable for freezing.

Barley Bread

4½ oz (127 g) sesame
  seeds
1 lb (454 g) barley
  flour
13 oz (368 g)
  wholewheat flour
2 oz (56 g) fresh yeast
1 pint 12 fl oz (9 dl)
  water
14 oz (397 g) plain
  white flour
4 tbsp
  polyunsaturated oil

Roast the sesame seeds in a dry frying pan until they begin to jump and pop. Roast the barley flour in the same fashion, stirring continuously until brown. Mix the sesame seeds, barley flour and wholewheat flour in a large mixing bowl. Dissolve the yeast in lukewarm water, and pour this over the flours. Stir until the batter is smooth and allow to rise about 30 minutes. Add the flour, salt and oil and stir well until a thick dough forms. Work the dough on a floured bread board and divide it into two or three parts. Shape each part into a loaf or place in a greased bread form. Allow the loaves to rise for about 30 minutes and bake in a very moderate oven, 350°F or Gas No 3 (175°C) for about 40 minutes.

This recipe can be varied by allowing the batter to stand for 2-3 days until it sours. Follow the instructions in the same way, and you then have a delicious Sour Barley Bread.

Poppy Rolls

20-25 ROLLS
12 fl oz (3.4 dl)
  skimmed milk
5 tbsp
  polyunsaturated oil
2 oz (56 g) fresh yeast
¾ tsp salt
1 lb-1 lb 2 oz
  (454-510 g) flour
1 egg
2 tbsp poppy seeds

Heat the milk and oil in a pan until lukewarm. Crumble the yeast into a bowl and pour over the milk and oil. Stir to dissolve the yeast and add the salt. Stir in the flour and work until a smooth but rather soft dough results. Knead on a floured bread board and shape the dough into oblong rolls; place them on a baking sheet and allow to rise until they have doubled in size. Brush with a beaten egg, and sprinkle with the poppy seeds. Bake in a very hot oven, 500°F or Gas No 9 (260°C) for about 8-10 minutes.

White Bread

18 fl oz (5.1 dl) water
2 oz (56 g) fresh yeast
2 tbsp
  polyunsaturated oil
½ tbsp salt
3½ oz (99 g) wheat
  germ
1 lb 9 oz (7 hg) plain
  white flour

Follow the instructions for Rye Bread (see p.121), but bake the loaves in a hot oven, 440°F or Gas No 7 (225°C), for about 20-25 minutes.

Breakfast Rolls

24 ROLLS
2 lb (9 hg) plain white
  flour
3 oz (85 g) wheat bran
1 oz (28 g) fresh yeast
1 pint 1 fl oz (6 dl)
  water
2 tbsp
  polyunsaturated oil
1 tbsp salt
poppy or sesame seeds

Mix the flour with the wheat bran. Make a little 'yeast pot'
with about 3½ fl oz (1 dl) of lukewarm water and the
yeast (see the recipe for Country Bread, p.120). Let it stand
for about 90 minutes. Heat the oil, water and salt until
lukewarm. Pour it on the 'yeast pot' and work the dough
until smooth and shiny. Cover the bowl with a tea towel
and allow to rise for about an hour. Knead the dough on a
floured bread board and divide it into 3 parts. Roll out
each part into a rectangle about 4 by 20 inches. Cut each
rectangle into 8 strips and roll each strip up from the short
side. Place the rolls on a greased baking tray, cover with a
cloth and allow to rise for a further 30 minutes. Brush the
rolls with cold water and sprinkle with poppy or sesame
seeds. Bake in a very hot oven, 500°F or Gas No 9 (260°C)
for 10-12 minutes.
  Allow the baked rolls to cool under a tea towel.

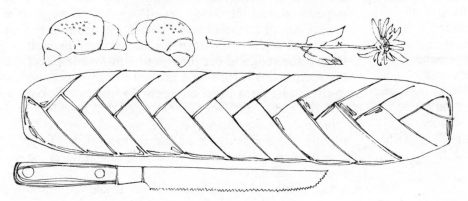

Hleb
Jugoslavian Bread

1 oz (28 g) fresh yeast
10½ fl oz (3 dl)
  mineral water
1 tsp salt
1 tbsp
  polyunsaturated oil
½ tsp baking soda
1 lb 2 oz (5.1 hg)
  plain white flour

Dissolve the yeast in lukewarm mineral water. Add the
salt, oil and baking soda. Stir in the flour a little at a time
and work the dough until smooth and shiny. Cover the
bowl with a tea towel and allow to rise for about 35
minutes. Place the dough on a floured bread board and
knead it. Cut the dough into 6 equal parts and roll each
one into a small ball. Place on a baking sheet and flatten
slightly. Cover with a tea towel and leave to rise for a
further 35 minutes. Prick the rolls with a fork several times
and fry them in a dry hot frying pan for a few minutes on
each side. After they have been browned slightly, place
them on a baking tray and bake in a very hot oven, 500°F
or Gas No 9 (260°C) for about 15 minutes. Let the rolls
cool slowly, wrapped in tea towels.

Tortillas (Mexican Flat Bread)

10 ½ oz (297 g) fine
ground maize flour
3 ½ oz (100 g) coarse
ground maize meal
¼ tsp salt
2 tbsp lemon juice
1 tbsp
polyunsaturated oil
8 ½ fl oz (2.4 dl) water

Mix flour, meal and salt in a large mixing bowl. Pour on the liquids and work the dough into a thick smooth consistency. Take small handfuls of the dough, work each into a ball, flatten it and roll it out with a rolling pin into a thin pancake about $\frac{1}{10}$-inch thick. Fry the tortillas in a hot dry frying pan, browning them on both sides.

Serve the tortillas as bread with meals or use them in various casseroles or other dishes.

Wholewheat Rusks

3 ½ fl oz melted high-
polyunsaturated
margarine
18 fl oz (5.1 dl)
skimmed milk
1 tsp salt
1 tbsp ground
cardamom
2 oz (56 g) fresh yeast
12 oz (340 g)
wholewheat flour
14 oz (397 g) plain
white flour

Mix together the margarine, milk, salt and cardamom. Dissolve the yeast in the lukewarm mixture. Add the flours and work the dough until smooth. Allow to rise for 25-30 minutes. Knead the dough on a floured bread board (the dough should be rather soft). Divide the dough into four parts, and work each part into a long sausage-like roll. Flatten the rolls and cut them into 2-inch-wide pieces. Place these small strips on a greased baking sheet and allow to rise under a tea towel for about 35 minutes. Bake in a very hot oven, 500°F or Gas No 9 (260°C) for 12-15 minutes. Remove them from the oven, allow to cool slightly and divide into tops and bottoms with a fork. Return them to the oven to roast the new surfaces for about 4-5 minutes.

Lower the oven temperature to an absolute minimum (as low as is possible with the oven still on), and allow the rusks to dry out thoroughly for at least 2 ½ hours.

Banana Bread

1 egg
3 ½ fl oz (1 dl)
skimmed milk
3 ½ tbsp high-
polyunsaturated
margarine
6 oz (170 g) plain
white flour
2 tsp baking powder
1 banana
3 egg whites

Beat the egg until foamy. Place the skimmed milk and margarine in a saucepan and heat until just short of boiling. Pour the liquid onto the beaten egg and stir. Mix the flour and baking powder together and stir this into the batter. Beat the egg whites very hard so that the tops will stand up by themselves, and fold this very gently into the batter. Bake in a very moderate oven, 350°F or Gas No 3 (175°C) for 45-50 minutes.

Index

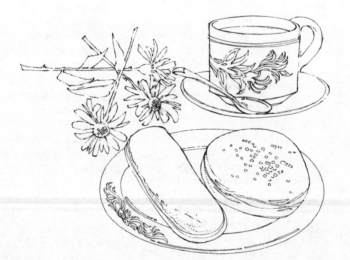